IT'S NOT THE CANS

The Best Nutrient Balance for a Stronger and Healthier You

BRYANT LUSK

To my wonderful mother, Dora Lusk. You are my
mentor, my hero, my dream come true.

To my fallen friends: Eric Roper, Harold F. Crawford, and Kenneth D.
Hunter. Our times together were cut far too short. I will never forget you.

Sincere Acknowledgments

To say "thank you" would be an understatement of my deeply felt appreciation for the people and organizations that enable me to push beyond perceived boundaries.

Claudia Vrinceanu provided a woman's perspective, which I so desperately needed. Her insights rounded out many of the rough edges that were apparent in the earlier drafts. She also loaned me her artistic eye to format the chapter titles and headings. This serves as further proof that I truly am from Mars.

Dr. Jesse McMullen PhD (FAA Technical Operations Training Division Manager) is a true inspiration to so many, yet he asks very little of so few. Jesse entrusted me to train and mentor thousands of Electronic Technicians and Engineers. Jesse's leadership empowered me with the knowledge, skill and ability to research, compile and organize information from a multitude of sources. I have rarely seen such strength of character, intellect, and authority displayed with such humility, sincerity and grace. Thank you Jesse, for who you are and for whom you have helped so many to become.

Finally, please allow me to express my sincere gratitude for the scientific organizations, government agencies, medical journals, medical professionals and nutrition experts throughout the world who created and distributed the raw data I used to support this work. These institutions and individuals work tirelessly to improve the health and wellbeing of us all. Their never ending contributions rarely make headlines but that does not diminish the very necessary and invaluable work they continue to perform on our behalf.

Contents

List of Tables

Introduction

I may be dating myself when I say *The Jerk*[1] is one of the funniest movies I have ever seen. It stars Steve Martin as Navin Johnson, a man going from rags to riches to rags. In one scene Navin works at a gas station with a sniper lurking nearby who is trying to shoot him. Fortunately, the sniper is a poor shot. He keeps missing Navin and hitting the oilcans next to him. As Navin watches the oilcans being hit, he puts two and two together and yells, "He hates these cans! Stay away from the cans!" As funny as that scene was, I never thought it could apply to real life. Based on the proliferation of faux diets today, it apparently does.

Faux is defined as "not genuine or intended to mislead." Faux diets are very misleading due to their reliance on ambiguous evidence and pseudoscience to support predetermined conclusions. Faux diets rarely disclose long-term health-risks associated with their weight management plans. In addition, they frequently promote an overly simplistic view toward nutrition to sell their agenda. To be fair, some faux diets do achieve short-term results. Unfortunately, they may come at a very high price, including vital nutrient deficiencies resulting in neurological disorders, hormonal imbalances, depressed immune response, bone loss (a contributor to osteoporosis), and heart disease.

Faux diets have flooded the internet with dangerous, health-related conclusions, similar to Navin's dangerous conclusion regarding the oilcans. Eventually, someone concerned with Navin's well-being helped him to recognize the cans were not the issue.

Much Better Than a Diet Plan

It's Not the Cans will enable you to recognize and address specific nutrient deficiencies that are often misdiagnosed and attributed to other health issues. These key nutrients play a vital role in your short-term and long-term health. Regardless of your age, gender, or level of fitness, nutrient balance can noticeably improve your health, weight, vitality, and overall performance. In addition, nutrient balance is much easier to achieve and maintain than some may realize.

It's Not the Cans also provides insight into the dangers and pitfalls of having excessive amounts of specific nutrients. Having too much of an individual nutrient can be just as damaging to your health and performance as having too little. Unlike faux diets, the information included here is based on credible, peer-reviewed, scientific studies independently conducted in multiple countries such as the United States, Canada, Japan, China, India, Germany, England, the Netherlands, Finland, Australia, South Korea, and others. In addition, information has not been cherry-picked to support foregone conclusions. A compilation of readily verifiable facts is the foundation upon which the conclusions are drawn.

Runners, weightlifters, cyclists, and couch potatoes alike can improve their health, focus, immunity, healing, and energy by reversing nutrient deficiencies and removing nutrient excess.

For example, many Americans are deficient in zinc, which can lead to many chronic health issues, including low testosterone. Low testosterone can trigger weight gain, muscle loss, fatigue, erectile dysfunction, and more. Zinc deficiency has also been linked to depression. The level of deficiency has been shown to directly correspond with the severity of some forms of depression.

Addressing a mild zinc deficiency alone can prevent and reverse a multitude of health issues. However, excessive zinc can lead to hypertension (high blood-pressure). Balance is key and it is achievable.

It's Not the Cans will empower you to understand, recognize, and reverse nutrient deficiencies and excesses that the majority of us do not even realize we have. Once you regain a nutrient balance, your cells will have the environment they need to maximize your strength, energy, metabolism, focus, performance, and overall health.

---

[1] Character name and quotations sourced from film "The Jerk" (1979). Aspen Film Society. William E. McEuen and David V. Picker Production.

My Story

I have worked in the field of aviation technology for nearly thirty years. As someone who is captivated by aviation, I never imagined that I would be fascinated by nutrients. Aviation technology excites me because it often delivers very remarkable results, such as making a 660,000-pound Boeing 777 aircraft that I just repaired defy gravity. Nutrients just didn't have the same "wow" factor for me—until now.

The Spark

My story began about two and a half years ago. It was a fairly normal day for me at work and at home. A few hours after going to bed, I woke up in excruciating pain. It was a foot cramp. Until that night, I had never suffered a foot cramp in my life and could not determine the cause. The very next evening, a new symptom arrived. As I lay quietly on my bed, I noticed that my heart was not beating at its normal pace. Whenever I took a deep breath, my heart appeared to pause. When I exhaled, my heart beat very rapidly for several seconds.

I decided to research my symptoms and potential treatment. I reviewed several data sources, such as WebMD, MedlinePlus, LiveStrong, and a host of other websites in search of reliable information about the cause of my condition. One constant that kept showing up was potassium. Based on what I read, low potassium seemed like a viable suspect. To verify my findings, I decided to see a physician. After I explained the reason for my visit, he listened to my heart and asked me to take a deep breath. I inhaled and held my breath, and my heart seemed to hesitate. He then asked me to release. I exhaled, and my heart raced for a few seconds.

After a moment, he looked at me and calmly said, "It may be your asthma. Asthma builds pressure in your chest, and that pressure may be affecting your heartbeat."

I explained that I'd had asthma for nearly forty years, and this condition had never happened before. I also pointed out that I was having foot cramps as well, which had never happened either.

I was given an EKG, and the results were normal. I asked, "Could it be low potassium?"

He told me that was rare and was most likely not the issue. I urged him to test my levels. He had my blood drawn, and my results came back as normal. That night, I suffered more foot cramps and the same sporadic heartbeat. Something had to give.

The Fire

I decided to take matters into my own hands and introduce potassium to my diet in a major way. I went online and downloaded a list of potassium-rich foods. I went to my local grocery store and purchased pomegranates, bananas, and cantaloupe. I also went to GNC and purchased potassium gluconate. I cut open the pomegranate and squeezed out as much juice as it would yield. I ate a banana and later took a couple of potassium pills (99 mg each) with my evening meal. That night, I still suffered a foot cramp, and my heart was still beating sporadically.

The next morning, I squeezed out another glass of pomegranate juice. I took a potassium pill with breakfast, lunch, and dinner. I also ate a banana and a section of cantaloupe. I did not have another foot cramp, and my heart maintained its natural rhythm. After a few days my symptoms were gone. I declared success! I was wrong.

The Cure

Seven months passed without incident. My feet were fine, and my heartbeat was solid as a rock. One night, in the middle of a very deep and restful sleep, I woke up in agony with a foot cramp. I couldn't believe it!

I decided to redouble my efforts to get an adequate amount of potassium each day. The nightly foot cramps continued. The only good news was that—despite the foot cramps—my heart was beating normally. Again, I did what researchers do and delved deeper into finding information about my symptoms. During my research, I noticed a recurring discussion of yet another mineral, magnesium.

Until then, I had never given magnesium much thought, especially as a nutrient. I discovered low magnesium could result in my symptoms. I also discovered just how critical this element was to numerous cellular functions and overall health. As I researched further, I was introduced to yet another nutrient called L-taurine. I had never heard of L-taurine in my life. So, I purchased magnesium and taurine supplements to add to my diet. Not only did my foot cramps completely subside, I also began to sleep much deeper and wake more rested. I regretted having allowed so many years to pass before becoming aware of the profound impact these nutrients have on my health.

The Journey

Throughout my career, I performed extensive research and analysis on extremely complex systems. When I realized that there was a lot about nutrients that I simply did not know, I leveraged my experience to research and analyze key nutrients and their impact on mental and physical health. In time, I found nutrient interaction to be just as fascinating as the aircraft, radar systems, and fiber-optic networks that I once worked on.

I began introducing various nutrient-rich foods and supplements to my diet. The next thing I knew, I had lost four pounds and looked noticeably leaner. This was totally unexpected, but it gets even better.

I have been using asthma inhalers for more than thirty years. Two months after I introduced key nutrients to my diet, I noticed that I was not using my rescue inhaler, Ventolin, as often. For the first time in years, I completely stopped using my preventive inhaler, Flowvent. I became so excited I began compiling and documenting nutritional data from around the world. *It's Not the Cans* was born.

Join me in a journey to identify key nutrient deficiencies that are often misdiagnosed—and never addressed. As stated earlier, regardless of your current level of health and fitness, the information that you are about to read can result in a leaner, stronger, and healthier you.

Are you ready? Then let us begin . . .

Good News

Despite day-to-day challenges, people today live longer than previous generations. During the period of 1980 to 2010, the centenarian population (persons 100 years of age or older) in the United States increased from 32,194 to 53,364 (65.8 percent), while the total United States population only increased 36.3 percent during the same period.[1]

In addition, average life expectancy has increased dramatically over the last century, from just 49 years at the turn of the twentieth century to just over 76 years by 1996. By 2008, white females (of Hispanic and non-Hispanic origin) maintained the highest life expectancy in the United States at 80.9 years, followed by black females at 77.2 years, white males at 76.1 years, and black males at 70.6 years.

Figure 1. Life Expectancy at Birth. United States, 1970–2009 [2]

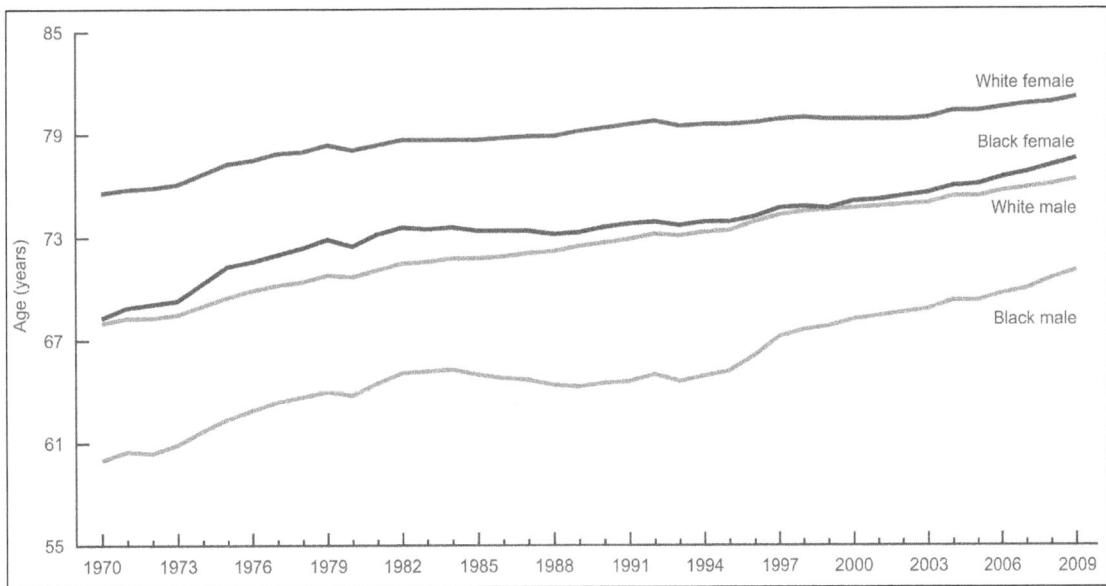

By 2009, we learned that in the United States, Hispanic females held the longest life expectancy at 83.5 years, followed closely by non-Hispanic white females at 81.1 years. Hispanic males came in third at 78.7 years, non-Hispanic black females came in at 77.4 years, non-Hispanic white males came in at 76.3 years, and non-Hispanic black male life expectancy was measured at 70.7 years (on average).

Figure 2. Life Expectancy at Birth. United States, 2006–2009 [2]

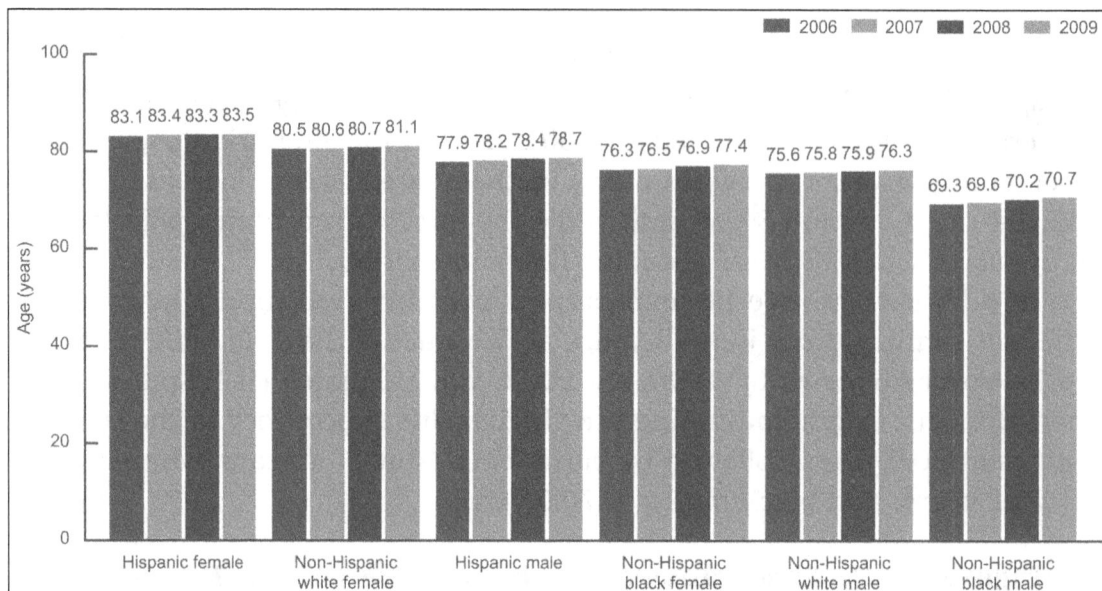

Figure 2. Life Expectancy at Birth. United States, 2006–2009 [2]

Legend: 2006 | 2007 | 2008 | 2009

Y-axis: Age (years)

Group	2006	2007	2008	2009
Hispanic female	83.1	83.4	83.3	83.5
Non-Hispanic white female	80.5	80.6	80.7	81.1
Hispanic male	77.9	78.2	78.4	78.7
Non-Hispanic black female	76.3	76.5	76.9	77.4
Non-Hispanic white male	75.6	75.8	75.9	76.3
Non-Hispanic black male	69.3	69.6	70.2	70.7

Although we are living longer, health is a growing concern. Many of us are lacking the nutrients our cells need to maximize health, focus, mood, and performance. Every action we take and decision we make begins at the cellular level. With improved cellular health, organs function better, the mind thinks more clearly, bones and muscles grow stronger, injuries heal more quickly, and we simply feel better.

Your cells need the proper balance of key nutrients for optimum performance. Let us begin our discussion with a remarkable nutrient that makes your bones and teeth stronger while preventing your arteries from hardening. You need only around 100 micrograms (mcg) a day, yet many people are deficient. This remarkable nutrient is called . . .

[1]   US Census Bureau, 2010 Census Special Reports, Centenarians: 2010, C2010SR-03
[2]   Arias E. United States life tables, 2009. National vital statistics reports; vol. 62, no 7. National Center for Health Statistics. 2014

Vitamin K2

Heart Disease, Bone Disease, Arthritis, Cancer,
Kidney Stones, and Tooth Decay

Vitamin K2 (a subcomponent of vitamin K) is required for healthy bones, teeth, and arteries. Just roughly 100 mcg of this amazing nutrient per day can reduce the calcium in your arteries (where you don't want it) and increase the calcium in your bones and teeth (where you do want it). Simply put, K2 prevents calcification (hardening) of the arteries and weakening of the bones and teeth. Without adequate K2 levels, the risk of stroke and cardiac arrest dramatically increases.

Vitamin K2 reduces arterial calcification by activating a matrix Gla-protein (MGP).[1] MGP protects the internal lining of your arteries from calcium deposits. In 2008 Dr. L.J. Schurgers et al. published a study [2] that states, "MGP is a potent inhibitor of arterial calcification." The study further points out that patients with cardiovascular disease had significant differences in MGP. Vitamin K2 is the catalyst for MGP activation.

Vitamin K2 activates another protein called Osteocalcin, which binds calcium to your bone tissue. In one study,[3] postmenopausal women were given MK-7 over a three-year period. MK-7 reduced age-related decreases in bone mineral density (BMD). In addition, MK-7 aided bone strength and significantly decreased the reduction of height (shrinkage) in the participants' vertebrae. An added benefit of this process is stronger teeth and potentially fewer cavities.

Vitamin K2 plays a preventive and therapeutic role in a variety of health issues.

Vegetarians

Unlike vitamin K1, vitamin K2 is naturally obtained through the consumption of animal-based products such as meats, cheeses, and eggs. This places vegans and vegetarians at a greater risk of developing vitamin K2 deficiency. Fortunately, K2 can be supplemented.

How Much and How Often

Vitamin K2 is available in two supplemental forms, synthetic MK-4 and natural MK-7. They both perform the same function. MK-4 dissipates from your blood serum within eight hours, whereas MK-7 is retained in your blood serum for up to seventy-two hours (three days). Also, it takes significantly higher supplemental doses of MK-4 to achieve similar results obtained through lower doses of MK-7. Due to its longer retention, natural formation, and ability to deliver results at lower doses, MK-7 may be the better option for supplementation. Nevertheless, additional data and more comparative studies are needed to make a definitive determination.

The total daily Adequate Intake (AI) for K2 is 90 mcg (micrograms) for women and 120 mcg (micrograms) for men. Studies concluded that higher intake of K2 resulted in lower mortality rates.[4] I do not endorse exceeding 200 mcg MK-7 or 5 mg of MK-4 in supplemental form per day unless directed to do so by a healthcare professional. Remember, you also obtain some K2 from food. Since a single dose of MK-7 remains active in your system for up to three days, it is perfectly fine to miss a day or two of supplementation. Long-term results may include stronger bones and teeth, fewer cavities, and a lower risk of osteoporosis, heart disease, and other illnesses. Many individuals are not likely to feel short-term results. Do not let that deter your efforts to achieve and maintain adequate (not excessive) levels. K2 is a marathon nutrient, not a sprint.

Although K2 appears to be safe at high doses, do not ingest excessive amounts. A small percentage of consumers have stated in online reviews that they have experienced elevated blood pressure and heart palpitations when initially taking K2 in the form of MK-7. A few consumers also stated that they had trouble sleeping when taking MK-7. The reviewers, however, did not indicate the amount (or dosage) that they ingested prior to these incidents occurring. You are encouraged to read reviews for the various brands that are available. Examine both good reviews and bad reviews to make an informed decision.

Vitamin K2 is a micronutrient. You only require a small amount for optimum bone and cardiovascular health. Therefore, supplement with caution. Additional details have been included in this chapter under the heading; *Listen to Your Body*.

Table 1. Vitamin K2—Food Type and Supplement Schedule

Food Type	When	How Often
natto (fermented soybeans) head cheese soft cheese egg yolks chicken breasts chicken livers	✓ With meals ✓ Between meals	❑ Any of these food items once or twice a day, 4 to 7 days per week Always consider fat, calories, and cholesterol intake.

Or Supplement

K2 as MK-7 (remains in your blood serum for up to 3 days)

Brand	When	How Often	
Nutrigold – Vitamin K2 MK-7 (100 mcg)	✓ With meals containing healthy fats (e.g., flaxseed, avocados, lake herring, lake trout, eggs, mackerel, wild salmon, tuna, sardines)	Loading phase	❑ 1 pill; mon, wed and fri ❑ Skip sat and sun ❑ 1 pill; mon, wed and fri ❑ Skip sat
		Maintenance phase	❑ 1 pill, 3 to 5 days per week (mon, wed, fri) (mon, tue, thr, fri) (any 5 days per week)
Now Foods MK-7 (100 mcg)	✓ Same as above	✓ Same as above	
Any reputable manufacturer	✓ Same as above	✓ Same as above (adjust for dosage)	

Absorption Inhibitors

Broad-spectrum antibiotics and medications used to lower cholesterol interfere with vitamin K. Excess vitamin A can inhibit the absorption of vitamin K. K2 is a sub-component of K.

Absorption Enhancers

Vitamin K2 is a fat-soluble nutrient. Taking a K2 supplement with a large or fatty meal increases its absorption. Foods with healthy fats such as eggs (cage-free), flaxseed (oil or milled), avocados, olive oil, lake herring, lake trout, mackerel, wild salmon, sardines, and tuna should be considered.

Preferred Product

Nutrigold MK-7 Gold. I purchase 120 softgels. By taking only three or four per week, one bottle provides an eight month supply.

Personal

Nutrigold MK-7 (100 mcg) K2 softgels are very small and look identical to vitamin D softgels. I alternate between taking one and two per day. I typically skip one or two day per week. As part of my normal diet, I receive additional K2 from eggs, cheese, and chicken.

Listen to Your Body

Several studies are available that list symptoms associated with vitamin K deficiency and excess. It is difficult to ascertain which, if any, of the information regarding vitamin K directly correlates to the subcomponent, vitamin K2.

Your body can convert vitamin K to its subcomponent, K2. Until recently, the lion's share of research has been on symptoms associated with vitamin K and K1. Now that K2 has been identified and made available as a supplement, more information is needed to help individuals differentiate symptoms of K2 deficiency and excess from symptoms associated with vitamins K and K1.

Warning

If you are taking blood-thinning medications such as Warfarin, do not take vitamin K supplements without consulting with your physician. As mentioned earlier, some consumers have stated in online reviews that they have experienced elevated blood pressure and heart palpitations when initially taking K2 in the form of MK-7.

Taking vitamin D and/or calcium supplements without having adequate levels of K2 may increase your rate of arterial calcification. Nevertheless, I strongly encourage you to ignore those who suggest consuming excessive amounts of vitamin K2 (or any nutrient). Balanced ratios are what your cells need to flourish.

Testing

The importance of this nutrient has only recently ascended to the nutritional spotlight. Therefore, it may be some time before reliable, verifiable testing methods are developed to measure K2 levels in individuals. Testing overall vitamin K levels is not an accurate indicator of vitamin K2 levels.

Very little vitamin K is stored in the body making direct measurement less than ideal. It has been suggested that a vitamin K2 assay test may be worth consideration. This test measures undercarboxylated osteocalcin as a functional marker of vitamin K2 levels. As discussed earlier, osteocalcin is a protein that is activated by the presence of vitamin K2.

Perform additional research before subjecting yourself to this or any other tests. Several unreliable sources of information have designed very impressive websites with scientific claims that are unproven. Proceed with caution.

Due to vitamin K2's effect on arterial calcification, you may also consider a coronary calcium scan[5] to monitor the health of your coronary arteries, and the effectiveness of your chosen brand of K2 supplements.

According to the National Heart, Lung, and Blood Institute (NHLBI), the coronary calcium scan looks for specks of calcium in the walls of the coronary arteries. Calcifications in the coronary arteries are an early sign of coronary heart disease (CHD).

[1] Beulens JW, Bots ML, Atsma F. Marie-Louise E.L. et al. (2008 Jul 07). High dietary menaquinone intake is associated with reduced coronary calcification. *Atherosclerosis*, 203, Issue 2, 489–493.

[2] Schurgers LJ, Cranenburg EC, Vermeer C. (2008 Sep 5). Matrix Gla-protein: the calcification inhibitor in need of vitamin K. *Thrombosis and Haemostasis*. 100(4):593-603. DOI: http://dx.doi.org/10.1160/TH08-02-0087

[3] Knapen MH, Drummen NE, Smit E, Vermeer C, Theuwissen E. (2013 Sep 24). Three-year low-dose menaquinone-7 supplementation helps decrease bone loss in healthy postmenopausal women. *Osteoporosis International*. (9):2499–507.

[4] Juanola-Falgarona M, Salas-Salvadó J, Martínez-González MÁ, et al. (2014 May). Dietary intake of vitamin K is inversely associated with mortality risk. The American Institute of Nutrition—Journal of Nutrition. 144(5):743-50.

[5] "What Is a Coronary Calcium Scan?" accessed July 18, 2014, http://www.nhlbi.nih.gov/health/health-topics/topics/cscan/

Zinc

Bone Health, Weight Loss, Cholesterol, Immune System,
Libido, Depression, Healing, Seizures, Asthma, ADHD,
Macular Degeneration, Muscle Cramps, Hair Loss, Acne

Zinc is one of several important minerals that are not receiving nearly the attention they deserve with regard to your mental and physical health. Many people are zinc–deficient without realizing it. It only takes a mild deficiency to have a major negative impact on your health.

Zinc plays a critical role in maintaining your immune system, metabolism, testosterone, mood, ability to heal, and more. In turn, these functions directly affect your weight, blood pressure, and energy. Retinal zinc concentrations decline as we age, which may affect eye health. In addition, overall zinc levels decline with age compromising immune function in the elderly.[1] Low zinc levels have been linked to diabetes.[2] Zinc has also been found to restore bone loss and increase bone mass.[3]

The brain contains the highest amount of zinc. Studies[4] show blood serum zinc levels to be low in people suffering from depression. In addition, the level of depression appears to correlate with the level of zinc deficiency. Zinc deficiency can also result in heightened aggression or violence. Elevated levels of copper can result from zinc deficiency, and trigger neurological disorders. In addition, lack of zinc can contribute to neuronal injury or death. One month supplementation of zinc gluconate resulted in a remarkable reduction in weight and BMI indices according to a 2013 research article in the Advanced Pharmaceutical Bulletin.[5]

Zinc is integral to natural testosterone production. Men and women need adequate testosterone levels to support numerous functions, including the growth and strength of healthy bones. Testosterone also helps men and women maintain muscle mass and healthy energy levels. Men and women with low testosterone may experience decreased libido, persistent fatigue, weight gain, a decreased sense of well-being, and more.

Unlike taking testosterone-enhancing drugs, attaining proper zinc levels does not introduce health risks. Testosterone-enhancers can increase your risk of heart attack, stroke, and mortality by nearly 30 percent. In one study,[6] total cholesterol levels increased 15 percent two days after a single testosterone injection. Proper zinc levels actually lower risk factors for additional health issues while improving your ability to naturally produce testosterone. Optimizing zinc intake could be a major step toward a healthier, and leaner you.

Vegetarians

The bioavailability (rate of absorption) of zinc from vegetarian diets is lower than from non-vegetarian diets.[7] Zinc contained in meat absorbs extremely well. In addition, vegetarians eat larger portions of foods that contain phytate. Phytate binds minerals such as zinc and strongly inhibits absorption. Vegetarians may require up to 50 percent more zinc than non-vegetarians to maintain adequate levels.

How Much and How Often

Zinc is an essential trace element. You require only low levels for optimum cellular performance. The RDA for zinc is 11 mg for men, and 8 mg for women. The daily Tolerable Upper Intake (UL) is 40 mg for men and women. If you are mildly to moderately zinc-deficient and increase your daily intake, you may begin to notice results in just one or two weeks. Results may include stronger libido, leaner muscle tone, and better performance at the gym. Long-term results may include faster healing of injuries, fewer illnesses, and healthier skin. Unlike other minerals, zinc cannot be stored in your body for later use. Consider eating zinc-rich foods or taking low-dose supplements at least three days per week.

Do not megadose on zinc. Studies[8] have shown that excessive zinc intake can cause a variety of neurological and physiological health problems, including high blood pressure. High blood pressure increases your risk of cardiac arrest and stroke. Continuous exposure to high levels of zinc can be extremely hazardous to your health.

Daily zinc intake of 40 mg or more can result in copper deficiency. Lower doses of zinc do not appear to diminish copper absorption. If you do not tolerate zinc well on an empty stomach, take it with a meal or try a different type.

Table 2. Zinc—Food Type and Supplement Schedule

Food Type	When	How Often
oysters, cooked (3 ounces)	✓ With meals ✓ Between meals	❑ Twice per week
beef chuck roast, braised (3 ounces), crab, Alaska king, cooked (3 ounces), beef patty, broiled (3 ounces), breakfast cereal, fortified with 25% of the DV for zinc (¾ cup serving)	✓ With meals ✓ Between meals	❑ Any of these food items once or twice per day, 4 or 7 days per week Always consider fat, calories, and cholesterol intake.

Or Supplement

Zinc monomethionine (absorbs extremely well; not easily impaired by phytate)
Zinc picolinate (absorbs extremely well; may irritate empty stomach)
Zinc citrate (absorbs well; may irritate empty stomach)
Zinc gluconate (absorbs well; may irritate empty stomach)

Brand	When	How Often	
Jarrow Formulas - Zinc Balance Zinc (15 mg) Copper (1 mg)	✓ Meals containing lean meat, fish, chicken, or eggs ✗ NOT with grains or dairy ✗ NOT with iron or calcium supplements	Loading phase	❑ 1 pill a day for 5 days ❑ Skip days 6 and 7 ❑ 1 pill a day for 5 days ❑ Skip days 13 and 14
		Maintenance phase	❑ 1 pill, 3 to 5 days per week (mon, wed, fri) (mon, tue, thr, fri) (any 5 days per week)
Solgar - Zinc Picolinate Zinc (22 mg)	✓ Same as above	✓ Same as above	

Absorption Inhibitors

Phytate, which is present in foods such as cereals, corn, and rice, inhibits zinc absorption. This does not suggest that these foods should be avoided. Avoid consuming foods high in phytate within 90 minutes of taking zinc supplements or eating zinc-rich meals.

Iron or calcium supplements, if taken together with zinc, can have a negative effect on zinc absorption. No effect on zinc bioavailability appears to occur from naturally occurring iron in a meal, such as within red meat. Some medications, such as antibiotics and diuretics, can also inhibit zinc absorption.

Foods that enhance zinc absorption counteract the effects of absorption inhibitors to some degree.

Absorption Enhancers

Meat-based protein such as beef, turkey, chicken, eggs, and seafood. These foods also help to counteract absorption inhibitors.

Preferred Product

Jarrow Formulas' Zinc Balance consists of zinc monomethionine and copper. The capsules are extremely small.

Personal

My total zinc intake consists of foods, Zinc Balance supplements, Solgar Zinc Picolinate (I cut the pills in half and alternate with Zinc Balance), and a dose of zinc contained in a daily multivitamin. I lost four pounds in one month after adding zinc supplementation and other key nutrients to my diet. In addition, after a month or so, use of my asthma rescue inhaler dramatically decreased (see *Nutrient-Based Remedies*).

Listen to Your Body

Symptoms of zinc deficiency can be easily misinterpreted or misdiagnosed. A compromised immune system resulting in frequent coughs or colds, sinus or respiratory infections, slow healing, and/or fatigue may be due to zinc deficiency. Mood swings, depression, ADHD, and difficulties with learning may also be symptoms of zinc deficiency. Zinc deficiency can trigger taurine deficiency (see *Taurine*) and/or low testosterone, which in turn may cause associated symptoms.

Very high levels of zinc can result in nausea, vomiting, loss of appetite, diarrhea, abdominal cramps, and/or headaches.

Megadosing on zinc will cause mineral imbalances, which can trigger mental and physical health problems. In addition, excessive zinc can cause hypertension (high blood pressure).

Warning

High-dose zinc intake greatly inhibits copper absorption and mildly inhibits iron absorption. You may also wish to consider slightly increasing iron intake via food or periodic supplementation (see *Iron*) when increasing zinc intake.

Testing

Zinc Taste Test may be an indicator of chronic zinc deficiency. Zinc sulphate is used for tasting and comparing the response. It is convenient yet very subjective.

Zinc Serum Test is more conventional. Unfortunately, several factors can cause inaccurate results.

Blood plasma can offer an estimate of zinc levels in tissue. Cell levels are more useful as a measure of zinc nutritional status.

Trial zinc supplementation at doses of 12–25 mg, four to five days per week, for a period of four to six weeks may reveal an existing zinc deficiency.

[1] Haase H, Rink L. (2009 June 12). The immune system and the impact of zinc during aging. *Immunity & Ageing.* 6: 9. doi: 10.1186/1742-4933-6-9.

[2] Singh RB, Niaz MA, Rastogi SS, Bajaj S, et al. (1998 Dec). Current zinc intake and risk of diabetes and coronary artery disease and factors associated with insulin resistance in rural and urban populations of *North India. Journal of the American College of Nutrition.* 17(6):564-70.

[3] Yamaguchi M. (2010 May). Role of nutritional zinc in the prevention of osteoporosis. *Molecular and Cellular Biochemistry.* 338(1-2):241-54. doi: 10.1007/s11010-009-0358-0.

[4] Swardfager W. Ph.D, Herrmann N. M.D., Mazereeuw G. Ph.D Candidate, et al (2013 Dec 15). Zinc in Depression: A Meta-Analysis. *Biological Psychiatry.* 74, (12): 872–878.

[5] Payahoo L, Ostadrahimi A, Mobasseri M, et al. (2013). Effects of Zinc Supplementation on the Anthropometric Measurements, Lipid Profiles and Fasting Blood Glucose in the Healthy Obese Adults. *Advanced Pharmaceutical Bulletin.* 3(1), 161-165. doi: http://dx.doi.org/10.5681/apb.2013.027

[6] Gårevik N, Skogastierna C, Rane A, et al. (2013 Dec). Single dose testosterone increases total cholesterol levels and induces the expression of HMG CoA reductase. *Substance Abuse Treatment, Prevention, and Policy.* 20(7):12.

[7] Foster M, Chu A, Petocz P, Samman S. (2013 Aug 15). Effect of vegetarian diets on zinc status: a systematic review and meta-analysis of studies in humans. *Journal of the Science of Food and Agriculture.* 93(10):2362-71.

[8] Kim J. (2013 Dec). Dietary zinc intake is inversely associated with systolic blood pressure in young obese women. *Nutrition Research and Practice.* 7(6):519.

Magnesium

*Blood Pressure, Heart Health, Weight Loss, Depression, Muscle Cramps,
Menstrual Cramps, Bone Health, Diabetes, Protein Synthesis, Migraines,
Sleep Disorders, Fatigue, ADHD, Kidney Stones, Nervous System*

Magnesium is an extremely important mineral. It is a key component to the health and performance of every bone, muscle, and organ in your body. Magnesium plays a vital role in regulating levels of other minerals such as calcium, potassium, zinc, and copper. Magnesium relieves and prevents muscle cramps and knots. It also helps maintain your sleep pattern and blood pressure.

Magnesium participates in the transport of potassium and calcium ions across your cell membranes for nerve impulse conduction, muscle contraction, and normal heart rhythm. It also normalizes your blood glucose levels. Magnesium is required to activate vitamin D, which enables you to absorb calcium. Magnesium is also an essential mineral for proper bone structure and density. As vital as magnesium is to mental and physical health, magnesium deficiency is common in the United States, especially among African Americans and the elderly.

Magnesium is necessary for many crucial metabolic functions, including DNA synthesis, protein synthesis, and neurotransmission. Studies identify magnesium deficiency as a risk factor for various forms of cancer, including breast cancer.[1] Magnesium is also associated with weight-loss.[2]

Magnesium deficiency appears to be linked to depression. According to one study,[3] "a variety of neuromuscular and psychiatric symptoms, including different types of depression, was observed in magnesium deficiency." A separate study [4] identified an inverse association between magnesium intake and depression. In other words, study participants with lower magnesium intake reported higher levels of depression.

Increased magnesium intake may lower the risk of sudden cardiac death (SCD).[5] In addition, dietary magnesium intakes roughly as high as 250 mg a day were associated with a significantly lower risk of ischemic heart disease caused by a reduced blood supply to the heart muscle [6].

The body stores almost half its magnesium inside the cells of tissues and organs. The other half is combined with calcium and phosphorus inside your bones. Less than one percent remains in your blood serum.

How Much and How Often

It can be challenging to obtain adequate amounts of magnesium through food alone. Foods containing the highest concentrations of magnesium such as almonds and spinach provide only about 20 percent of the RDA per serving. Given the average American diet, many people may have to supplement at least 50 percent of their daily magnesium requirements to maintain adequate levels. The percentage of supplementation requirements may increase with age due to decreased dietary intake and decreased absorption. This is especially true for older adults due to increased magnesium secretion via the urine.

Magnesium supplements come in various forms. Chelated magnesium glycinate, magnesium citrate, and a few others yield a very high level of bioavailability. The absorption rate of magnesium oxide is extremely low. Approximately four percent is absorbed. Unfortunately, many popular multivitamin brands contain magnesium oxide.

The RDA for magnesium is 310–320 mg (for women) and 400–420 mg (for men). Yet, the daily Tolerable Upper Intake Level (UL)—the level at which a person may possibly suffer mild stomach or intestinal upset—is 350 mg for women and men. A body-weight method suggests the average person should consume roughly 2.7–3 mg of magnesium for every pound of body-weight. A 130-pound person would consume 350–390 mg. These figures reflect your total intake from all sources, not just from supplements.

If you are magnesium deficient, you should notice results within two days to two weeks. Results may include fewer or less severe muscle cramps and muscle knots, deeper sleep, diminished menstrual cramps, and more. Long-term results may include improved heart function, better insulin regulation, stronger bones and teeth, and improved mineral utilization.

You do not need excessive doses to achieve results. Both low and excessive magnesium levels can have significant, long-term harmful effects on your bone health. If you increase your magnesium intake yet still suffer from symptoms of deficiency, low potassium is an area worth exploring. The vast majority of us are chronically low in potassium. This is especially true for individuals who regularly engage in high-intensity physical activity.

Although low magnesium levels can trigger other nutrient deficiencies, megadosing on magnesium will not offset deficiencies in nutrients that are the result of inadequate intake. Identifying and maintaining the proper intake range of vitamins and minerals is integral to a healthy future.

Table 3. Magnesium—Food Type and Supplement Schedule

Food Type	When	How Often
almonds, dry roasted, 1 ounce spinach, boiled, ½ cup cashews, dry roasted, 1 ounce peanuts, oil roasted, ¼ cup soymilk, plain or vanilla, 1 cup black beans, cooked, ½ cup edamame, shelled, cooked, ½ cup peanut butter, 2 tablespoons bread, whole wheat, 2 slices avocado, cubed, 1 cup	✓ With meals ✓ Between meals	❏ Any of the food items, 5 to 8 times a day, 5 to 7 days per week Always consider fat, calories, and cholesterol intake.

Or Supplement

Chelated buffered magnesium glycinate (absorbs extremely well)
Chelated magnesium citrate (absorbs well)

Brand	When	How Often	
Swanson – Buffered Chelated Magnesium Glycinate (133 mg) or Swanson – Time Released Buffered Chelated Magnesium Glycinate (200 mg)	✓ With meals ✓ Between meals ✓ After workout ✓ Prior to sleep ✓ With meals ✗ NOT with calcium, caffeine, or grains	Maintenance phase (only)	❏ 1 to 2.5 mg per pound of your body weight, 5 to 7 days per week Do not exceed 400 mg in a single dose.
Transdermal Magnesium • magnesium bath additive • magnesium oil spray • magnesium lotion • magnesium gel	✓ As directed	Maintenance phase (only)	❏ As directed by the product label

Absorption Inhibitors

Calcium strongly inhibits the absorption of magnesium. Magnesium absorption decreases as we age. Foods high in phytate or oxalates, such as grains, bran, un-sprouted beans, soy, spinach, leafy greens, nuts, tea, coffee, and cacao also inhibit absorption. Try not to consume these foods within 90 minutes of taking magnesium supplements.

Calcium, iron, copper supplements, and mineral-rich foods should be consumed separately from magnesium for maximum absorption. Alcoholic beverages, soda, stress, bleached sugar, intense workouts, and diabetes deplete magnesium.

Magnesium oxide has an extremely low absorption rate and should not be counted toward your daily intake.

Absorption Enhancers

Vitamin D enhances magnesium absorption. Complex carbohydrates, protein (other than soy), and medium chain triglycerides (MCTs), such as coconut oil and palm oil enhance the absorption of magnesium.

Preferred Product

Swanson's Buffered Chelated Magnesium Glycinate is an extremely high-quality magnesium that is very affordable when purchased from the company's website. Other reputable manufacturers may also be considered.

Personal

My daily magnesium intake consists of magnesium-rich foods and a Swanson Buffered Chelated Magnesium Glycinate supplement. I supplement with 266–399 mg of magnesium every day. I take one capsule with dinner and two additional capsules prior to going to bed.

I stopped having foot cramps the first night that I took magnesium supplements. In addition, use of my asthma rescue inhaler drastically decreased within a month of including potassium and zinc supplementation taken separately (see *Nutrient-Based Remedies*).

Listen to Your Body

Symptoms of magnesium deficiency include depression, anxiety, hypertension, muscle cramps, muscle knots, sensations of numbness or tingling, irregular heartbeat, loss of appetite, nausea, fatigue, sleep disorders, severe menstrual cramps, seizures, memory lapses, hallucinations and/or disorientation.

High doses of magnesium supplements may result in diarrhea, nausea, and/or abdominal cramping.

Warning

Drinking excess water increases the depletion rate of magnesium. If you regularly drink several glasses of water, ensure that you replenish your magnesium stores via foods or supplements. Do not ingest excessive amounts of magnesium in a single day.

Testing

Blood serum tests for magnesium levels can be extremely inaccurate.

Recognizing symptoms, sublingual epithelial cell analysis, diet assessment, or trial supplementation may be required to ascertain the likelihood and severity of an existing magnesium deficiency

A sublingual epithelial cell analysis for magnesium is considered to be more accurate than blood serum tests.[7]

You are encouraged to perform additional research before subjecting yourself to any testing procedure. For more information, please visit www.notthecans.com/info/.

[1] Ko HJ, Youn CH, Kim HM, et al. (2014 Jun) Dietary Magnesium Intake and Risk of Cancer: A Meta-Analysis of Epidemiologic Studies. *Thyroid Research Journal.* 9:1-9.

[2] Dean C. (2012 Jun 3). Magnesium - The Weight Loss Cure. *Natural News.* http://www.naturalnews.com/036049_magnesium_weight_loss_cure.html

[3] Serefko A, Szopa A, Wlaź P, et al. (2013) Magnesium in depression. *Pharmacological Reports.* 65(3):547-54.

[4] Jacka FN, Overland S, Stewart R, et al. (2009 Jan) Association between magnesium intake and depression and anxiety in community-dwelling adults: the Hordaland Health Study. *The Australian and New Zealand Journal of Psychiatry.* 43(1):45-52. doi: 10.1080/00048670802534408.

[5] Peacock JM, Ohira T, Post W, Sotoodehnia N, et al. (September 2010 Sep). Serum magnesium and risk of sudden cardiac death in the atherosclerosis risk in communities. (ARIC) Study. *American Heart Journal.* 160(3):464-4–70.

[6] Del Gobbo LC, Imamura F, Wu JH, et al. (2013 Jul). Circulating and dietary magnesium and risk of cardiovascular disease: a systematic review and meta-analysis of prospective studies. *The American journal of clinical nutrition.* 98(1):160-73. doi: 10.3945/ajcn.112.053132.

[7] Haigney MC, Silver B, Tanglao E, et al. (1995 Oct 15) Noninvasive Measurement of Tissue Magnesium and Correlation with Cardiac Levels. *Circulation.* 92(8):2190-7.

Vitamin D3

*Cancer, Diabetes, Osteoporosis, Depression, Weight Loss,
Dementia, Alzheimer, Blood Pressure, Multiple Sclerosis,
Autoimmune Diseases, Mortality, Heart Health, Flu*

According to the National Institutes of Health,[1] vitamin D "is a fat-soluble vitamin naturally present in very few foods, added to others, and available as a dietary supplement. It is also produced endogenously when ultraviolet rays from sunlight strike the skin and trigger vitamin D synthesis. Fortified foods provide most of the vitamin D in the American diet. In the 1930s, a milk fortification program was implemented in the United States to combat rickets. Both the United States and Canada mandate the fortification of infant formula with vitamin D."

Many individuals are aware of vitamin D's role in bone health and the prevention of osteoporosis. What may come as news to some is the fact that calcitriol, the active form of vitamin D, is actually a hormone that is needed to support many biological functions to include hormone production. It also provides protection against colon, prostate, and breast cancer. In addition, vitamin D is vital for proper immune function.[2] 1,200 IU of vitamin D3 supplementation has even been shown to prevent respiratory infections and the flu.[3]

Vitamin D deficiency has been linked to obesity[4] and several chronic illnesses. A large cohort study[5] associated vitamin D deficiency with all-cause mortality, cardiovascular diseases, cancer, and respiratory diseases. Vitamin D deficiency is also linked to significantly greater risk of dementia and Alzheimer disease.[6]

Magnesium activates vitamin D inside your system. Low magnesium can result in low serum levels of vitamin D. In addition, vitamin D can increase the rate of hardening of the arteries if adequate vitamin K2 levels are not maintained. Nutrient balance is essential.

Vitamin D stores extremely well in your body's fatty tissue. Skin exposure to direct sunlight for fifteen minutes six days in a row can provide enough vitamin D for several weeks. Certain ethnic groups, such as African Americans, require longer exposure to obtain the same levels.

Vitamin D supplementation comes in two forms; ergocalciferol (D2) and cholecalciferol (D3). Multiple studies[7],[8] have concluded that vitamin D2 should no longer be used as a supplement or for fortification purposes. In addition, D3 is more effective than D2 at raising serum 25(OH)D (vitamin D) concentrations. The human body is much more compatible with D3.

How Much and How Often

Current RDA values for vitamin D are 600 International Units (IU) for everyone except children younger than twelve months old (400 IU) and adults older than seventy-one (800 IU). These values represent the total intake throughout the day from multiple sources, not from a single food or supplement. Mounting evidence suggests that the RDA for vitamin D is too low for optimum health. It appears that 8,400-14,000 IU per week (an average of 1,200-2000 IU a day) is an adequate target range until further studies are conducted.

Some have taken the extreme view of suggesting daily doses as high as 10,000 IU. Unfortunately, high levels of vitamin D can raise serum calcium levels, which leads to vascular and tissue calcification and subsequent damage to the heart, blood vessels, and kidneys.[9]

Our bodies are extremely efficient at storing vitamin D. The daily Tolerable Upper Intake Levels (UL) for vitamin D is 4,000 IU per day. If you are vitamin D–deficient, regaining proper levels should yield results within a few weeks (decreased muscle cramps, improved sleep, and a more positive outlook). Long-term results should include stronger teeth and bones, and a noticeably improved immune system.

Magnesium deficiency can potentially manifest itself as a vitamin D deficiency. As mentioned in the previous chapter, blood serum tests for determining true magnesium levels are very unreliable.

Current protocol for addressing a diagnosed vitamin D deficiency consists of administering 50,000 IU of D2 in a single dose. Even though multiple studies (cited previously) concluded that vitamin D2 should no longer be used, this protocol is still in practice today.

As treatment for a medically-diagnosed vitamin D deficiency, a daily regimen of 300 to 500 mg of highly-bioavailable magnesium in conjunction with 5,000 to 10,000 IU D3 should be considered. Said treatment would be administered in place of current D2 protocol.

In order to mitigate the risk of arterial calcification, 90 to 150 mcg of vitamin K2 (MK-7) should be considered in conjunction with treatment. A reduction of daily calcium supplementation should also be considered if it exceeds 500 mg. This is mainly due to the restoration of D3, magnesium and K2 levels, which should significantly enhance calcium absorption and utilization.

This information should not be viewed as medical advice. Rather, these are points to consider discussing with your physician if you have questions regarding vitamin D deficiency.

Table 4. Vitamin D3—Food Type and Supplement Schedule

Food Type	When	How Often
cod liver oil, 1 tablespoon (1,360 IU) swordfish, cooked, 3 ounces (566 IU) salmon (sockeye), cooked, 3 ounces (447 IU)	✓ With meals ✓ Between meals	❑ Any of these items once a day Always consider fat, calories, and cholesterol intake.

Or Supplement		
Vitamin D3 (absorbs extremely well)		

Brand	When	How Often
Nutrigold D3 (2,000 IU)	✓ Meals containing healthy fats (e.g., flaxseed, olive oil, avocados, lake herring, lake trout, mackerel, wild salmon, eggs, sardines, tuna)	Loading phase: ❑ 2 softgels a day for 5 days ❑ Skip days 6 and 7 ❑ 2 softgels a day for 4 days ❑ Skip days 12, 13 and 14 Maintenance phase: ❑ 1 softgel, 3 to 4 days per week or 2 softgels, 2 days per week (mon, thr) (mon, wed, fri) (mon, tue, thr, fri)
Nutrigold D3 (5,000 IU)	✓ Same as above	Loading phase: ❑ 1 softgel a day for 5 days ❑ Skip days 6 and 7 ❑ 1 softgels a day for 4 days ❑ Skip days 12, 13 and 14 Maintenance phase: ❑ 1 softgel, 2 days per week (mon, thr)

Absorption Inhibitors

Sunscreen impedes vitamin D production. Conditions that affect digestion can reduce vitamin D absorption. Kidney disease, and certain medications also inhibit the absorption of vitamin D.

UVB radiation does not penetrate glass. Therefore, glass between your skin and sunlight prevents vitamin D synthesis from occurring.

Absorption Enhancers

Vitamin D is a fat-soluble nutrient. Taking vitamin D3 with a meal significantly increases absorption. Vitamin D3 is more effective at increasing serum levels when not taken every day. Smaller doses (2,000 IU or less) are absorbed more fully than larger doses. Magnesium activates vitamin D after the vitamin D has been absorbed.

Preferred Product

Nutrigold D3 is natural, sourced from lanolin, encapsulated in organic olive oil, and GMO free. It is available in doses of 1,000, 2,000, and 5,000 IU. Other reputable manufacturers such as NOW Foods are also worth considering.

Personal

My weekly dietary intake of vitamin D typically falls between 9,100–14,000 IU. I consume one Nutrigold D3 softgel (2000 IU) three days per week and one or two Citracal-Petites, five or six days per week. I also enjoy Horizon Organic low-fat milk, meals, and sunshine.

Listen to Your Body

Symptoms of vitamin D deficiency may compromise the immune system resulting in frequent coughs and colds, sinus or respiratory infections, slow healing, and/or fatigue. Vitamin D deficiency may also present itself as poor bone and teeth density and structure.

When levels of vitamin D become too high, signs of toxicity include nausea, vomiting, poor appetite, constipation, weakness, and weight loss. By raising blood levels of calcium, too much vitamin D can cause confusion, disorientation, and problems with heart rhythm.

Warning

Taking vitamin D supplements without adequate vitamin K2 may increase risk for developing cardio vascular disease (see *Vitamin K2*).

African Americans, nightshift workers, and seniors should have their vitamin D levels tested more frequently than other individuals.

High serum levels of vitamin D are associated with greater risk of cancer at some sites such as the pancreas, greater risk of cardiovascular events, and more falls and fractures among the elderly.

Testing

The Vitamin D Council [10] (VDC) lists three ways to get tested:

1. Ask your doctor for a vitamin D test. Be specific and ask for a 25(OH) D test. The 25(OH)D test is the only one that will tell you whether you're getting enough vitamin D.
2. In-home tests are sent to your residence. You prick your finger and put a drop of blood on to some blotter paper. You send the paper to a laboratory to be tested. Companies that offer in-home tests, include:
   - ZRT Labs. The Vitamin D Council works with ZRT Labs.
   - Century Diagnostics via Home Health Testing.
   - City Assays. Based in the UK and offers the cheapest test internationally. It takes about 10 days for the test to arrive to the USA.
3. Order a test online and get blood work done at a laboratory.

[1]   "NIH Vitamin D Fact Sheet for Health Professionals," last reviewed June 24, 2011, http://ods.od.nih.gov/factsheets/VitaminD-HealthProfessional/.

[2]   Aranow C. (2011 Aug) Vitamin D and the Immune System. *J Investig Med.* 59(6): 881–886. doi: 10.231/JIM.0b013e31821b8755.

[3]   Urashima M, Segawa T, Okazaki M, et al. (2010 May) Randomized trial of vitamin D supplementation to prevent seasonal influenza A in schoolchildren. *The American Journal of Clinical Nutrition.* 91(5):1255-60. doi: 10.3945/ajcn.2009.29094.

[4]   Rock CL, Emond JA, Flatt SW, et al. (2012 Nov). Weight loss is associated with increased serum 25-hydroxyvitamin D in overweight or obese women. *Obesity (Silver Spring, Md.).* 20(11):2296-301. doi: 10.1038/oby.2012.57.

[5]   Schöttker B, Haug U, Schomburg L, et al. (2013 Apr) Strong associations of 25-hydroxyvitamin D concentrations with all-cause, cardiovascular, cancer, and respiratory disease mortality in a large cohort study. *Rev Med Interne.* 97(4):782-93. doi: 10.3945/ajcn.112.047712.

[6]   Littlejohns T, Henley W, Lang IA, et al. (2014 Aug 6) Vitamin D and the risk of dementia and Alzheimer disease. *Neurology.* 29(10):815-20. doi: 10.1212/ WNL.0000000000000755.

[7]   Mistretta VI, Delanaye P, Chapelle JP, et al. (2008 Oct) Vitamin D2 or vitamin D3. *Rev Med Interne.* 29(10):815-20. doi: 10.1016/j.revmed.2008.03.003.

[8]   Houghton LA, Vieth R. (2006 Oct). The case against ergocalciferol (vitamin D2) as a vitamin supplement. *The American Journal of Clinical Nutrition.* 84(4):694-7.

[9]   "NIH Vitamin D Fact Sheet for Health Professionals", accessed July 24, 2014, http:// ods.od.nih.gov/factsheets/VitaminD-HealthProfessional/

[10] "Testing for vitamin D," accessed July 16, 2014, http://www.vitamindcouncil.org/ about-vitamin-d/testing-for-vitamin-d/.

Taurine (L-Taurine)

Weight Loss, Diabetes, Anxiety, Blood Pressure, Sleep Disorders, Eye Health, Epilepsy, Longevity, Brain Function, Depression, Congestive Heart Failure, Anti-Neurotoxic, Tumors, Liver Function, Tinnitus

Taurine is a very basic amino acid that plays a critical role in supporting and maintaining numerous biological functions at the cellular level. It is one of the most plentiful amino acids in the brain, retina, muscle tissue, and organs. Taurine plays a positive role in weight loss, diabetes, anxiety, sleep disorders, congestive heart failure, and much more. Evidence indicates taurine lowers blood pressure and calms the sympathetic nervous system. Taurine contributes to the normal brain development of the fetus and newborn babies. In addition, taurine deficiency was found to be more prevalent in autistic children [1].

Taurine improves muscle endurance and metabolizes fat (especially belly fat). In one double-blind randomized study [2], taurine significantly reduced body weight in comparison to the participants who were given a placebo. In addition, in 2010, a six week anti-obesity study [3] conducted on rodents resulted in significantly lower weight gain with taurine added to the diet.

Taurine promotes deeper and more sustainable sleep, especially when taken in conjunction with 200—400 mg of chelated magnesium glycinate or citrate. Foods containing taurine are red meat, seafood, milk, and eggs.

A 2010 study [4] conducted by Yukio Yamori, et al concluded:

> World-wide epidemiological studies conducted for the last 25 years revealed that 24U-T [taurine] was inversely associated with the age-adjusted mortality rates of stroke and CHD [coronary heart disease]. High 24U-T, particularly combined with high M [magnesium] excretion, was associated highly significantly with lower CVD [cardio vascular disease] risks, obesity, hypertension, hypercholesterolemia and AI [atherogenic index]. These findings indicate the consistency of the beneficial T effects on animal models and humans proven either experimentally or epidemiologically. Such consistency of the extensive basic and epidemiological findings of T effects

and the effects combined with M indicates greater prospective for T [taurine] to contribute to the nutritional prevention of CVD and lifestyle-related diseases.

Vegetarians

Taurine is primarily an animal-based amino acid. Vegetarians may be chronically deficient in taurine. Lack of taurine associated with a meat-free diet can result in mood swings and other issues related to anxiety.[5] Fortunately, taurine can be safely and affordably supplemented.

How Much and How Often

Taurine appears to be safe at high levels. Good results seem to occur within a daily intake the range of 500–2,000 mg. Though there is no RDA for taurine at this time, there appears to be little to no added benefit from exceeding 3,000 mg per day. Please keep in mind that individuals do obtain some taurine from animal products. In addition, taurine is produced naturally in the body.

Do not exceed 2,000 mg of supplemental taurine per day unless directed to do so by a physician. Also consider cycling this product by taking it four or five days on, two or three days off, or take it every other day. Many people do not cycle taurine and may not agree.

If you are taurine-deficient, you may notice results within two days to two weeks. Short-term results may include deeper sleep (especially when taken with magnesium) and more energy. There are simply too many potential long-term positive results associated with taurine to list here. Please search "taurine benefits" on any reputable search engine for more detailed information.

Table 5. Taurine—Food Type and Supplement Schedule

Food Type	When	How Often
whole capelin (6,174 mg) cooked Dungeness crab (5,964 mg) Alaskan salmon fillets (4,401 mg) lamb (3,676 mg)	✓ With meals ✓ Between meals	❏ Any of these items every other day Always consider fat, calories, and cholesterol intake.

Or Supplement		
Taurine capsules or tablets (absorbs extremely well)		

Brand	When	How Often
Solgar – Taurine (500 mg)	✓ With meals ✓ Between meals ✓ Prior to sleep	Maintenance phase (only	❏ 1 or 2 capsules, 4 to 6 days per week (mon, wed, fri) (mon, tue, wed, thr) (any 5, or 6 days)
Jarrow Formulas – Taurine (1,000 mg)	✓ Same as above	Maintenance phase (only)	❏ 1 capsule, 4 to 6 days per week (mon, wed, fri) (mon, tue, thr, fri) (any 5, or 6 days)
Any reputable manufacturer	✓ Same as above	✓ Same as above (adjust for dosage)	

Absorption Inhibitors

Monosodium glutamate (MSG) may inhibit taurine absorption and/or production. Anaerobic bacteria (anaerobes) inhibit taurine production. Vitamin A, zinc, or vitamin B6 deficiency also reduces natural taurine production.

Food, in general, may retard taurine absorption to some degree as taurine is absorbed during direct contact with the lower intestine. However, I suggest taking it with a protein-rich meal in order to reduce the risk of developing peptic ulcers and acid reflux.

Absorption Enhancers

As an amino acid, taurine is readily absorbed. Your body's natural taurine production is enhanced by vitamin A, D3, and zinc.

Preferred Product

Jarrow Formulas (1,000 mg) and Solgar (500 mg) taurine. Any reputable manufacturer may be considered.

Personal

As a stand-alone supplement, 1,000 mg of taurine made me a little sluggish when taken during the day. I also found it slightly more difficult to maintain intensity and focus during my workouts unless I included an energy enhancer such as C4 Extreme. I have since ceased taking taurine during the day.

I currently take 500–1,000 mg of Solgar taurine four or five nights per week with dinner, followed by 233–400 mg of magnesium before going to bed. I no longer awaken in the middle of the night with an inability to go back to sleep. I have more frequent, memorable dreams. I have not slept this deeply—or dreamed this vividly—in nearly twenty years.

Listen to Your Body

Low levels of taurine may present itself in the form of low muscle mass, obesity, anxiety, seizures, varied neurological disorders,[6] hypertension, poor heart function, gout, lower than optimum endurance, and/or impaired vision.

Warning

High doses of taurine can increase stomach acid levels, which can result in heartburn and peptic ulcers.

There is one report of brain damage in a bodybuilder who took nearly 14 grams of taurine (14,000 mg) along with insulin and steroids. It is not known which, if any, of the substances caused the injury.

In addition, a consumer reported having a noticeable impairment to short-term memory after taking taurine. The short-term memory returned to normal after ceasing taurine supplementation.

Testing

Taurine levels can be measured via urine analysis. In addition, measuring taurine levels in whole blood may yield more accurate results than measuring levels contained within blood plasma.

[1]   Pangborn J. (2002) Autism: metabolic differentiation, role of DPPIV/CD26, some pertinent lab tests. In: Rimland B, ed. DAN! (Defeat Autism Now!) Spring 2002 Conference. San Diego, CA: *Autism Research Institute.*

[2]   Zhang M, Bi LF, Fang JH, et al. (2003 Dec 15). Beneficial effects of taurine on serum lipids in overweight or obese non-diabetic subjects. *Amino Acids.* 26 (3): 267–71. doi: 10.1007/s00726-003-0059

[3]   Du Hl, You JS, Zhao X, et al. (2010 Aug 24). Antiobesity and hypolipidemic effects of lotus leaf hot water extract with taurine supplementation in rats fed a high fat diet. *Journal of Biomedical Science.* 17(Suppl 1):S42. doi: 10.1186/1423-0127-17-S1-S42.

[4]   Yamori Y, Taguchi T, Hamada A, et al. (2010 Aug 24). Taurine in health and diseases: consistent evidence from experimental and epidemiological studies. *Journal of Biomedical Science.* 17 Suppl 1:S6. doi: 10.1186/1423-0127-17-S1-S6. http://www.jbiomedsci.com/content/17/S1/S6

[5]   Laidlaw SA, Shultz TD, Cecchino JT, et al. (1988 Apr) Plasma and urine taurine levels in vegans. *The American Journal of Clinical Nutrition.* 47(4):660–3.

[6]   Perry TL, Bratty PJ, Hansen S, et al. (1975 Feb) Hereditary mental depression and Parkinsonism with taurine deficiency. *Archives of Neurology.* 32(2):108-13.

Potassium

*Stress, Irregular Heartbeat, Heart Attack, Cancer, Insulin
Resistance, Menopause, Insomnia, Infant Colic, Allergies,
Headaches, Acne, Alzheimer's, Arthritis, Vision, Bloating,
Fever, Gout, Irritability, Muscle Weakness, Muscular Dystrophy,
Chronic Fatigue, Intestinal Disorders, Dermatitis*

Potassium is an electrolyte that is vital for life. The vast majority of people rarely meet the necessary daily requirements. The more active you are, the more potassium you need to replenish your supply. It plays a critical role for every cell in your body. Potassium is required for key cell functions, such as nerve impulse conduction, normal heart rhythm, and blood glucose levels. It is also required to build muscle and to burn carbohydrates for energy. Potassium is essential for all of your muscle contractions, including cardiac, skeletal, and smooth muscle tissue.

Potassium actively lowers blood pressure in people who suffer from hypertension (high blood pressure).[1],[2] Hypertension dramatically increases your risk factor for cardiac arrest and stroke. Potassium intake is directly associated with bone mineral density (BMD). Research [3] indicate that individuals with higher potassium intake maintain greater BMD, thus reducing their risk of developing osteoporosis.

Health issues associated with sodium often result from an extremely low intake of potassium. Potassium helps you expel sodium via your urine. Of the various supplemental forms, potassium citrate is alkaline, potassium gluconate is pH neutral, and potassium chloride is acidic (see "pH balance" in the Glossary of Terms). Your kidneys regulate potassium levels by excreting it through the urine. Drinking excess water depletes your potassium via urination.

Potassium citrate prevents and reduces kidney stones by adhering to calcium in the urine. Potassium citrate also prevents the urine from becoming too acidic. Potassium gluconate may be the better option absent underlying health issues, such as kidney stones.

Low-carb diets place individuals at greater risk for developing a potassium deficiency.

How Much and How Often

The daily adequate intake (AI) recommendation is 4,700 mg for adults, which roughly equates to twelve bananas per day. Low-sodium V8 and pure coconut water are excellent sources of potassium.

Supplemental potassium can be found in tablet, capsule, and powder forms. Potassium pills are regulated not to exceed 99 mg of elemental potassium. This is due to high concentrations (in pill form) irritating and/ or damaging portions of the stomach lining by remaining in direct contact for extended periods. Powdered potassium, when added to liquid, is safe at higher doses than pill form.

According to a five year NHANES study [4] (2005–2010) comprised of 10,563 participants, the usual intakes of sodium and potassium were 3,569 mg/day (sodium) and 2,745 mg/day (potassium), reflecting a dietary ratio of 1.41:1. Based on this study, many adults need to consume an additional 40 percent (1,880 mg) of the recommended AI to maintain proper levels of potassium for optimum health. This number is even higher for individuals that drink a lot of water or engage in various forms of exercise.

Supplemental potassium should always be taken with a meal or directly after to protect the stomach lining and induce a slower, even absorption rate. If you weigh 160 pounds or more, I encourage you not to exceed 400 mg (powder) in a single dose. I encourage individuals weighing less than 160 pounds to not exceed 2.3 mg (powder) for each pound of bodyweight in a single dose. For instance, an individual who weighs 130 pounds would not exceed (roughly) 300 mg (2.3 mg X 130) in a single dose unless directed to do so by a physician. You may choose to take two to four separate doses a day.

Always consider that many stand-alone supplemental nutrients are absorbed more rapidly, and more completely than food-based nutrients. For instance, 800 mg of potassium contained in two bananas does not absorb in the same manner as 800 mg of pure supplemental potassium, which in a single dose can be extremely dangerous, especially if consumed on an empty stomach. Potassium is used by your body to make your muscles contract. Your heart is a muscle.

If you are potassium-deficient, you may notice results within two days to two weeks, including fewer muscle cramps, a more relaxed respiratory system, and more endurance during physical activities. Long-term results could include improved weight management, lower blood pressure and improved heart function.

A combination of potassium-rich foods and beverages coupled with periodic supplementation can help individuals reach and maintain healthy potassium levels.

Table 6. Potassium—Food Type and Supplement Schedule

Food Type	When	How Often
low-sodium V8 pure coconut water potatoes (baked) sweet potatoes (baked) spinach squash pure pomegranate juice (not from concentrate)	✓ With meals ✓ Between meals	❑ Any of these food items 3 times a day
baked beans bananas orange juice cantaloupe tuna milk	✓ With meals ✓ Between meals	❑ Any one of these food items 2 times a day in addition to potassium supplementation Always consider sugar intake.

Or Supplement

Potassium gluconate powder (absorbs well with food; mild taste of potassium)
Potassium gluconate pills (absorbs well; 99 mg each)

Brand	When	How Often	
NOW – Potassium Gluconate Powder (270 mg elemental potassium)	✓ With meals (add to beverage of choice)	Maintenance Phase (only)	❑ 400 to 800 mg, 5 to 7 days per week in 2 or more separate doses
Any reputable manufacturer – Potassium Gluconate Pills (99 mg elemental potassium)	✓ With meals	Maintenance Phase (only)	❑ 3 or 4 pills per day, 5 to 7 days per week in 3 or 4 separate doses

Absorption Inhibitors

Alcoholic beverages and caffeine inhibit potassium absorption. More importantly, they cause your kidneys to flush additional potassium out of your system via the urine. Drinking large amounts of water will also deplete your potassium stores due to increased urination. Low magnesium levels may increase potassium secretion from your body.

Apples, cabbage, grapes, green beans, and plums contain low levels of potassium and therefore should be replaced with foods containing higher concentrations.

Absorption Enhancers

Potassium is absorbed extremely well within your lower intestines.

Preferred Product

NOW's Potassium Gluconate Powder (270 mg per serving) may be added to water, juice, milk, or smoothies. NOW's Potassium Gluconate Pills (99 mg) is also a good product that may be taken with each meal. NOW's
Potassium Citrate is another good option, especially for those who suffer from kidney stones. Any reputable manufacturer will suffice.

Personal

My initial daily supplementation fell between 700–900 mg via potassium gluconate powder. I replaced supplemental potassium with potassium-rich foods and beverages such as Low Sodium V8. Each glass contains a whopping 900 mg of potassium. Each 11.5 oz. can contains 1,180 mg. Each 5.5 oz. can contains 700 mg.

Listen to Your Body

Low potassium can result in a variety of symptoms such as; muscle—cramps, twitches, or weakness—fatigue, low energy, abnormal heart rhythm, tingling or numbness sensations, confusion, depression, psychosis, delirium, and in some cases, hallucinations.

Excessive potassium levels (hyperkalemia) can be extremely hazardous to your health. Symptoms include muscle fatigue, weakness and paralysis, abnormal heartbeat and cardiac arrest.

Individuals with healthy kidneys rarely experience issues from supplemental potassium.

Warning

When consuming adequate amounts of potassium, the human body is very efficient at managing excess via the kidneys. Nevertheless, impaired kidney function such as with diabetics, can generate dangerously high levels of potassium.

Potassium deficiency can also be a symptom of magnesium deficiency. In addition, drinking excess water increases the depletion rate of potassium and magnesium. If you drink a lot of water, ensure that you replenish your potassium and magnesium stores.

Testing

Blood serum tests for potassium levels are a poor indicator for actual tissue levels. Tissue releases it stores of various nutrients in order to maintain proper levels in the blood.

A sublingual epithelial cell analysis 5 may be considered for measuring potassium levels within your tissue. The test kit is shipped to your local physician who collects small soft-tissue samples from the mouth.

You are encouraged to engage in additional research before subjecting yourself to any testing procedure. For more information, please visit www.notthecans.com/info/.

[1] Haddy FJ, Vanhoutte PM, Feletou M. (2006 Mar) Role of potassium in regulating blood flow and blood pressure. *American Journal of Physiology. Regulatory, Integrative and Comparative Physiology.* 290(3):R546-52.

[2] He FJ, Markandu ND, Coltart R, et al. (2005 Apr). Effect of short-term supplementation of potassium chloride and potassium citrate on blood pressure in hypertensives. *Hypertension.* 45(4):571-4.

[3] Tucker KL, Hannan MT, Chen H, et al. (1999 Apr). Potassium, magnesium, and fruit and vegetable intakes are associated with greater bone mineral density in elderly men and women. Am J Clin Nutr. 69(4):727-36.

[4] Zhang Z, Cogswell ME, Gillespie C, Fang J, Loustalot F, et al. (2013) Association between Usual Sodium and Potassium Intake and Blood Pressure and Hypertension among U.S. Adults: NHANES 2005–2010. PLoS ONE 8(10): e75289. doi:10.1371/journal.pone.0075289

[5] "Magnesium and Heart Disease", accessed August 27, 2014, http://www.exatest.com/

Iodine

*Metabolism, Fatigue, Depression, Immune System,
Cancer, Fibrosis, Testosterone, Cholesterol, Coronary
Artery Disease, Autoimmune Diseases, Hair Loss*

Iodine is a trace element that is essential for proper thyroid function. Thyroid hormones regulate many important biochemical reactions and are critical for metabolic activity. Iodine also shrinks cancer cells and causes apoptosis (automatic cell death) of some cancer cells. Chlorine and fluoride, contained in municipal drinking water, inhibit iodine absorption. Iodine deficiency during early childhood is a major cause of brain impairments throughout the world.

A 2009 study in Switzerland [1] indicates that roughly half of the European population is mildly iodine deficient. A 2008 United States Food and Drug Administration (FDA) Total Diet Study [2] indicates that iodine intake levels in the United States ranged from 138 to 353 mcg per day.

Vegetarians

Vegetarians and vegans are at greater risk of developing iodine deficiency than others. Soy and cruciferous vegetables, such as cabbage, broccoli, cauliflower, and Brussels sprouts, interfere with the utilization of iodine. [3]

How Much and How Often

The RDA for iodine in adults is 150 mcg. The upper limit is approximately 1 mg (1000 mcg). In the event of a radiological incident, the CDC recommends a single dose of 130 mg of potassium iodide for adults under forty years of age.

Attaining proper iodine levels can yield short-term and long-term benefits. People who are extremely deficient may see results within a few weeks, such as increased energy and weight loss. If you are not deficient, you may not feel any results. Positive results may occur very gradually over several months for mild iodine deficiencies.

A few people have ignited an iodine megadosing frenzy suggesting supplementation of up to 12.5 mg per day. They may unknowingly cite a 1967 research paper focused on iodine consumption in Japan.

A 2005 editorial in the Townsend Letter[4] suggests the belief that people in Japan consume 13.8 mg of iodine a day may have resulted from a study conducted in 1967.[5] The editorial indicates that the study found Japanese seaweed consumption (on average) to be 4,600 mg a day. The seaweed contained 0.3% iodine. 4,600 mg multiplied by 0.003 gives you 13.8 mg of iodine. However, the calculation used wet seaweed, which added water weight. Actual seaweed weighs much less. Regrettably, many who have bought into magadosing iodine are unaware of this. By measuring iodine intake via urinary excretion, studies[6] found iodine intake among Japanese people ranging from 330–470 mcg per day.

Moreover, in 2011, Theodore T. Zava and David T. Zava performed a comprehensive review of iodine intake in Japan by measuring seaweed consumption [7]. The study indicates that, Kombu seaweed, which has the highest iodine content in Japanese seaweed, loses as much as 99 percent of its iodine after it is boiled fifteen minutes. The study concluded, that the average Japanese iodine intake is 1,000–3,000 mcg per day, which is far short of the 12,500 mcg megadosers recommend.

When you factor in foods that block iodine absorption such as the variety of cruciferous vegetables within the Japanese diet, the amount of iodine absorbed is even less. In addition, bromide concentrations among people in Japan [8] are fairly high and directly blocks iodine absorption.

Even though the majority of credible data does not support taking large amounts of iodine, megadosers suggest taking gradually increasing amounts to build a tolerance. Doing so will cause the thyroid to decrease its iodine absorption rate and your kidneys to eliminate more iodine via urine. Building a tolerance to iodine is counterproductive to your health and your wallet.

Anyone in the United States who may need additional iodine will likely only require an additional average daily intake of 30–100 mcg. This can easily be achieved via slight changes to one's diet such as the use of iodized salts or low-dose, periodic supplementation. Women who are pregnant require more iodine than they would otherwise need.

China's National Iodine Deficiency Disorders Elimination Program [9] decreased goiter rates among children from 20.4 percent to 8.8 percent in four years via iodized salt. The International Council for the Control of Iodine Deficiency Disorders (ICCIDD) Global Network [10] and the American Thyroid Association [11] confirm that 150 mcg of iodine is adequate for most adults (with the exception of pregnancy).

Table 7. Iodine—Food Type and Supplement Schedule

Food Type	When	How Often
sea vegetables cod turkey breast eggs milk yogurt cranberries navy beans potatoes (baked)	✓ With meals ✓ Between meals	❑ Any of these food items 2 or 3 times a day

Or Supplement		
Nascent (atomic) iodine (absorbs exceptionally well; superior form of iodine) Molecular iodine (absorbs well on empty stomach) Potassium iodide (absorbs moderately well)		

Brand	When	How Often
LL -Magnetic Clay Nascent Iodine - 1 Oz (400 mcg per drop)	✓ Between meals with water	Maintenance Phase (only) ❑ 1 drop, 1 to 3 days per week (mon, thr) (mon, wed, fri)
Go Nutrients – Iodine Edge Nascent Iodine (~300 mcg per drop)	✓ Between meals with water	Maintenance Phase (only) ❑ 1 drop, 1 to 3 days per week (mon, thr) (mon, wed, fri)
NOW – Kelp Caps (150 mcg)	✓ Meals containing lean meat, fish, chicken, or eggs	Maintenance Phase (only) ❑ 1 pill, 2 to 4 days per week (mon, thr) (mon, wed, fri) (mon, tue, thr, fri)

Absorption Inhibitors

Fluoride; chlorine; bromide (bromine, bromate) found in white flour, breads, rolls, and soda inhibit the thyroid's ability to absorb iodine. Soy, and cruciferous vegetables such as cabbage, broccoli, cauliflower, and Brussels sprouts interfere with iodine absorption. Caffeine products may also inhibit iodine absorption. Try not to consume these products within 60 minutes before or 30 minutes after taking iodine supplements or eating iodine-rich foods.

Absorption Enhancers

Nascent (atomic) iodine absorbs extremely well on an empty stomach. Directions for use typically require the consumer to add a drop of liquid iodine to a glass of water and swallow. Nascent iodine can also be absorbed sublingually. It has been reported to be less toxic and better tolerated than other forms. There is no risk of heavy metals.

Molecular iodine supplements have grown in popularity and appear to absorb well on an empty stomach. Be advised that some forms of molecular iodine are sold in extremely high doses.

Potassium iodide is primarily absorbed within the GI tract and is considered less effective than nascent iodine. With the exception of a properly diagnosed medical condition, a daily (or every other day) regimen of 50 to 150 mcg should serve to maintain your thyroid health.

Preferred Product

Iodized salt is very useful for maintaining proper iodine levels. LL's Magnetic Clay Nascent Iodine (atomic iodine) is extremely effective.

Personal

I maintain iodine levels via multivitamins and diet. I enjoy iodine-sourced foods such as cage-free eggs, salmon, tuna, and more. My average daily intake is roughly 240 mcg, far short of the 12.5 mg that megadosers recommend. I am happy, healthy and energetic.

Listen to Your Body

Iodine deficiency can cause impaired mental function, fatigue, goiter, or hypothyroidism (underactive thyroid). With hypothyroidism you may feel colder, suffer memory lapses or depression. Detailed symptoms are listed under *Hashimoto's Disease* starting on the following page.

Severe iodine deficiency during pregnancy can result in children with mental and growth disorders.

Excessive iodine can cause autoimmune disease, and/or thyroid cancer from long-term exposure. It can also cause hypothyroidism, or hyperthyroidism (overactive thyroid) resulting in nervousness, irritability, anxiety, difficulty sleeping, perspiration, rapid heartbeat, hand tremors, brittle hair and muscle fatigue.

Warning

On June 5, 2013, the American Thyroid Association [12] released a statement advising against the daily ingestion of iodine supplements in excess of 500 mcg. They further state that consuming more than 1,100 mcg of iodine per day may cause thyroid dysfunction. In addition, some iodine supplements derived from kelp may contain heavy metals.

Supplement iodine with extreme caution. Your thyroid gland directly impacts every aspect of your health and fitness.

Testing

Urine analysis for iodine excretion levels is very common. Blood serum analysis, however, may yield more accurate results.

Due to iodine characteristics and various environmental factors, I remain skeptical about the validity of iodine skin tests as an indicator for iodine deficiency. Additional testing methods are available.

Hashimoto's Disease

As stated by the Office on Women's Health [13], Hashimoto's disease (Hashimoto's thyroiditis) is an autoimmune disease that affects the thyroid. Thyroid hormone levels are controlled by the pituitary gland inside the brain. It makes thyroid-stimulating hormone (TSH), which triggers the production of thyroid hormone. With Hashimoto's disease, the immune system makes antibodies that damage thyroid cells and interfere with their ability to make thyroid hormone. Excessive iodine can trigger Hashimoto's thyroiditis in people prone to getting it.

Over time, thyroid damage can cause thyroid hormone levels to be too low (hypothyroidism). An underactive thyroid causes every function of the body to slow down, including heart rate, brain function, and the rate your body turns food into energy. Hashimoto's disease is the most common cause of an underactive thyroid. It is closely related to Graves' disease, another autoimmune disease affecting the thyroid.

Many people with Hashimoto's disease have no symptoms for years. An enlarged thyroid, called a goiter, is often the first sign of disease. It rarely causes pain.

Hashimoto's disease is about seven times more common in women than in men. It can occur in teens and young women, but more commonly shows up in middle age. Many people with Hashimoto's disease may have mild or no symptoms at first. But symptoms tend to worsen over time. Symptoms of an underactive thyroid include:

- Fatigue
- Weight gain
- Pale, puffy face
- Feeling cold
- Joint and muscle pain
- Constipation

- Dry, thinning hair
- Heavy menstrual flow or irregular periods
- Depression
- A slowed heart rate
- Problems getting pregnant

[1] Zimmermann MB. (2009 May). Iodine Deficiency. *Endocrine Reviews*. 30(4):376-408

[2] Murray CW, Egan SK, Kim H, Beru N, et al. (2008 Nov) US Food and Drug Administration's Total Diet Study: dietary intake of perchlorate and iodine. *J Expo Sci Environ Epidemiol*. 18(6):571-80. doi: 10.1038/sj.jes.7500648.

[3] Krajcovicová-Kudláčková M, Bucková K, Klimes I, et al (2003 Sep). Iodine Deficiency in Vegetarians and Vegans. *Nutrition & Metabolism*. (47):183–185

[4] "Iodine: A Lot to Swallow", published Sept 2005, http://www.townsendletter.com/AugSept2005/gabyiodine0805.htm

[5] Nagataki S, Shizume K, Nakao K. (1967 May 1) Thyroid function in chronic excess iodide ingestion: comparison of thyroidal absolute iodine uptake and degradation of thyroxine in euthyroid Japanese subjects. *J Clin Endocrinol Metab*. (27):638–647. doi: http://dx.doi.org/10.1210/jcem-27-5-638.

[6] Ishizuki Y, et al. (1994 Dec 20) The variation of Japanese urinary excretion of iodine in different decades of age. *Nippon Naibunpi Gakkai Zasshi*. (70):1093–1100

[7] Zava T, Zava D. (2011 Oct 5) Assessment of Japanese iodine intake based on seaweed consumption in Japan: A literature-based analysis. *Thyroid Research Journal*. (4):14.

[8] Zhang ZW1, Kawai T, Takeuchi A, et al. (2001 May) Urinary bromide levels probably dependent to intake of foods such as sea algae. *Archives of Environmental Contamination and Toxicology*. 40(4):579-84.

[9] Delange F1, Bürgi H, Chen ZP, et al. (2002 Oct). World status of monitoring iodine deficiency disorders control programs. *Thyroid*. 12(10):915-24

[10] "FAQs about Iodine Nutrition." Accessed September 3, 2014, http://www.iccidd.org/p142000264.html

[11] "Iodine Deficiency", published June 4, 2012, http://www.thyroid.org/iodine-deficiency/

[12] "ATA Statement on the Potential Risks of Excess Iodine Ingestion and Exposure," June 5, 2013, http://www.thyroid.org/ata-statement-on-the-potential-risks-of-excess-iodine-ingestion-and-exposure/

[13] "Hashimoto's disease fact sheet", last updated July 16, 2012, http://womenshealth.gov/publications/our-publications/fact-sheet/hashimoto-disease.html

Iron

*Fatigue, Immune System, Anemia, Metabolism, Tissue
Formation, Depression, Wound Healing*

Iron is an essential nutrient for transporting oxygen throughout your body. It is also crucial to cell growth and differentiation. A deficiency of iron can lead to fatigue, decreased immunity, or a consistent feeling of being cold. The two forms of iron in our diets are heme (from meat) and nonheme (from plants). Heme iron is more readily absorbed and is not easily impeded by other foods. Nonheme iron is less efficient than heme iron and is easily impaired by other foods. Iron absorption increases when body stores are low and decreases when stores are high.

According to the World Health Organization (WHO)[1], iron deficiency is significantly prevalent in industrialized countries.

As much as 80 percent of the world's population may be mildly to severely iron-deficient. Using its three possible classifications—mild, moderate, and severe—the WHO classified iron deficiency in the United States as a "moderate" public health problem. Iron deficiency occurs gradually. The need for iron may be as high as 30 percent greater for individuals who engage in intense exercise on a regular basis. Female athletes, distance runners, and vegetarian athletes are at greater risk of being iron deficient.

Vegetarians

Nonheme iron absorption is readily impaired by phytate, which is typically found in legumes and whole grains. Soy-based protein also impedes nonheme iron absorption. Vegetarians who exclude all animal products from their diets may need almost twice as much dietary iron each day as non-vegetarians because of the lower intestinal absorption of nonheme iron in plant foods. Vegetarians should consider consuming nonheme iron sources together with a good source of vitamin C.

How Much and How Often

Supplemental iron is available in two forms: ferrous and ferric. Ferrous iron salts (ferrous fumarate, ferrous sulfate, and ferrous gluconate) appear to be the best-absorbed forms of supplements.

The RDA for iron is only 8 mg for males nineteen and older. The RDA is 18 mg for females from the ages of nineteen to fifty (27 mg if pregnant), and only 8 mg for females fifty-one and older. The daily tolerable upper intake for iron is 45 mg for males and females eighteen years of age or older.

The average person expels or depletes approximately 1 or 2 mg of iron per day. There is no need to take iron every day. If you are iron-deficient, you should notice results after several weeks (increased energy, more stamina, better focus, warmer body temperature, fewer illnesses, and improved healing).

Iron can be taken as a stand-alone supplement or it may be included in a daily multivitamin. No one should need to supplement 100 percent of their iron requirements, this is especially true for non-vegetarians. Daily, low-dose supplementation or moderate doses taken twice per week should suffice. Excess iron can be extremely hazardous to your health.

Women who are very active or experience heavy menstrual bleeding should closely monitor their iron levels. Vegans, athletes and individuals who take mineral supplements should also monitor their iron levels more closely than others. Consult with your physician.

If taking a multivitamin containing iron, additional iron supplementation may not be warranted.

Before considering iron supplementation, it is wise to have your iron levels tested. In addition, consider getting tested for genetic disorders such Glucose-6-Phosphate Dehydrogenase (G6PD) deficiency. G6PD deficiency occurs more often in males and mainly affects red blood cells. The most common medical problem associated with G6PD deficiency is hemolytic anemia, which develops when red blood cells are destroyed more quickly than the body can replace them. Individuals of African, Asian or Mediterranean descent are more prone to having this genetic disorder than others. G6PD deficiency tends to be more severe among individuals of Mediterranean origin.

People with Northern European ancestry are more prone to a genetic disorder called Primary Hemochromatosis (iron overload) and should consider being tested for it prior to iron supplementation.

According to the National Heart, Lung and Blood Institute (NHLBI)[2], some people with primary hemochromatosis do not suffer from associated health issues, even with high levels of iron in their bodies. Some individuals have severe complications and can even die from the disease. The severity of the disease can be affected by other factors such as high intake of vitamin C, which increases the severity of the disease.

See the paragraph entitled *Listen to Your Body* for more details.

Table 8. Iron—Food Type and Supplement Schedule

Food Type	When	How Often
meat fish poultry spinach kale broccoli beans lentils	✓ With meals ✓ Between meals	❏ Any food item 2 or 3 times a day Always consider fat, calories, and cholesterol intake.
Or Supplement		
Heme iron (absorbs extremely well; not readily impaired by absorption inhibitors) Nonheme iron (absorbs okay; readily inhibited by foods and minerals)		
Brand	**When**	**How Often**
GNC – Gentlesorb Iron (18 mg)	✓ Between meals ✓ Meals containing lean meat, fish, chicken, or eggs ✗ NOT with grains or dairy ✗ NOT with zinc or calcium supplement	Women Maintenance Phase (only) ❏ 1 capsule, 1 to 3 days per week (mon, thr) (mon, wed, fri) Men Maintenance Phase (only) ❏ 1 capsule, 1 to 2 days per week (sun, wed)
Solgar - Gentle Iron Bisglycinate (25 mg)	✓ Same as above	✓ Same as above
Lactoferrin	✓ As directed	✓ Same as above (adjust for dosage)
Any reputable manufacturer	✓ As directed	✓ Same as above (adjust for dosage)

Absorption Inhibitors

According to the CDC,[3] the absorption of iron supplements can be inhibited if taken with calcium. Iron absorption is also inhibited by tannins in coffee or tea, dairy, eggs, oxalic acid-spinach, kale, beets, nuts, chocolate, tea, wheat bran, rhubarb, strawberries, herbs-oregano, basil, and parsley and phytate (grains and legumes). Heme iron is not as susceptible to absorption inhibitors as nonheme iron.

Absorption Enhancers

Vitamin C is often recommended to enhance iron absorption. However, one study[4] indicates that taking iron and ascorbic acid together can cause ulcers, and can potentially lead to cancer. Taken iron and vitamin C separately do not generate the same risk. Meat-based protein also enhances iron absorption.

Preferred Product

GNC's Gentlesorb iron has should not upset the stomach therefore can be taken with or without a meal. Solgar is another gentle product. Perform additional research to find the iron that works best for you.

Personal

I chose to supplement with GNC's Gentlesorb iron at 18 mg per capsule. I mainly eat grilled chicken breasts, turkey, tuna, and baked salmon. I eat steak or brisket once per week. I also eat a lot of dark, leafy salads that include romaine lettuce, broccoli or kale.

I have G6PD. I only take supplemental iron once per week.

Listen to Your Body

According to the Iron Disorders Institute, "People with iron disorders can have many vague symptoms or health issues including any one or combination of the following: fatigue, joint pain, bone or joint disease (osteoarthritis, osteoporosis), shortness of breath, irregular heartbeat, liver trouble, diabetes, infertility, impotence, depression, mood or mental disorders, poor cognitive skills or neurodegenerative diseases."

The Iron Disorders Institute further suggests a person can be iron deficient and not anemic. In addition, a person can have "false anemia" such as when fighting off harmful bacteria.

On the other hand, hemochromatosis (iron overload) occurs when excess iron builds up in the blood and organs, such as the liver and heart. As stated previously, primary hemochromatosis is a genetic trait. People of Northern European descent are more prone to hereditary hemochromatosis. Secondary hemochromatosis can be caused by an illness or excessive iron supplementation. Hemochromatosis may go undiagnosed until an organ is damaged. Symptoms include fatigue, weakness, weight loss, abdominal pain, and joint pain. If you suffer from any symptoms, see a doctor immediately.

Warning

Blood loss—including menstrual bleeding—accelerates the depletion of iron. If you have not had your iron levels tested in the past three years, consider doing so.

In children, death has occurred from ingesting 200 mg of iron. It is important to keep iron supplements tightly capped and out of children's reach.

Iron supplementation can be hazardous to individuals with:

- G6PD deficiency
- Hemochromatosis

Testing

According to the Iron Disorders Institute, iron is tested in a variety of ways to determine different functions:[5]

Serum Iron (SI)
Total Iron Binding Capacity (TIBC)
Transferrin-iron Saturation percentage (TS%)
Serum Ferritin (SF)
Hemoglobin (Hgb)

Please visit Iron Disorders Institute's website for more details at: http://www.irondisorders.org/iron-tests/

[1]   "Micronutrient deficiencies: Iron deficiency anaemia," accessed July 17, 2014, http://www.who.int/nutrition/topics/ida/en/.
[2]   "What Is Hemochromatosis?", accessed September 1, 2014, http://www.nhlbi.nih.gov/health/health-topics/topics/hemo/.
[3]   "Iron and Iron Deficiency," accessed July 18, 2014, http://www.cdc.gov/nutrition/everyone/basics/vitamins/iron.html.
[4]   Fisher AEO, Naughton D. (2004 Jan 16). Iron supplements: the quick fix with long-term consequences. Nutrition Journal. 3: 2. doi:10.1186/1475-2891-3-2.
[5]   "Iron Tests," accessed July 18, 2014, http://www.irondisorders.org/iron-tests/.

Calcium

Bone and Teeth Health, Heart Health, Nervous System, Blood Clotting

Calcium supports a wide variety of cellular activities. Almost all calcium is stored in bones and teeth, where it supports their structure and hardness. The body also needs calcium for muscle movement, for normal heart function, and to allow nerves to transmit messages between the brain and the rest of the body.

Before your body can utilize calcium, you need proper levels of vitamin D to absorb it. Before vitamin D can effectively help you absorb calcium, you need proper levels of magnesium to activate vitamin D. Magnesium is also a major component inside your bone structure. Once calcium is absorbed, it needs a guide to direct it to your bones and teeth. Without a guide, calcium builds up inside your arteries over time, making blood circulation more difficult—even to the point of cardiac arrest. Vitamin K2 is that guide (see *Vitamin K2*).

If you regularly consume calcium-rich foods or supplements and are diagnosed with calcium deficiency, low magnesium is a potential suspect. The same is true of vitamin D. As stated in a previous chapter, low magnesium levels can contribute to vitamin D deficiency. This then leads to poor calcium absorption.

As the title *It's Not the Cans* suggests, a calcium deficiency may not be the result of something as obvious as low calcium intake. In such cases, taking more calcium to reverse a calcium deficiency may not be effective, and could even be counterproductive to your long-term health. It may be prudent to examine the first "domino" in the calcium utilization sequence and work your way forward to determine where the calcium supply line may have been compromised. One should first start a journal to document what they eat. Document every food and beverage consumed each day for one week. Go to notthecans.com/info and follow the Diet Assessment link to determine your nutrient intake.

The concentration of calcium in the body tends to decline as we age. In addition, as women age, absorption of calcium may decline due to reduced estrogen levels. Deficiencies in nutrients such as vitamin D, iodine, or zinc affect estrogen production. Again, always consider going back to the first step in the process and working your way forward to identify the issue versus only addressing the symptom. Calcium absorption can vary depending on race, gender, and age. Lowering calcium intake does not appear to prevent kidney stones. Potassium citrate does prevent and dissolve kidney stones (see *Potassium*).

How Much and How Often

Calcium supplements come in various forms. Calcium carbonate requires stomach acid to be absorbed and must be taken with a meal. Calcium citrate, which can be more expensive, is more readily absorbed (with or without food). My only concern with calcium carbonate is that calcium (in any form) impedes the absorption of other minerals. Therefore, taking calcium with a meal increases the risk for key mineral deficiencies. When possible, calcium supplements and calcium-rich foods should be consumed outside of major meals and mineral supplementation for more effective mineral absorption.

Concerns have been raised over the levels of heavy metals, such as lead and mercury, contained in coral calcium. A study[1] on calcium supplements found concentrations of lead at 0.106-0.384 mg/kg in oyster, coral and animal bone, which are considered natural-raw calcium. Traces of mercury and cadmium were also detected. Lead was not found in calcium gluconate or calcium citrate.

If you choose to supplement with coral calcium or a similar product, purchase from a reputable manufacturer. In addition, ensure the product has been tested for heavy-metals and other hazardous elements. The RDA for elemental calcium varies with age.

Males and females ages 19 to 50 (1,000 mg)
Males ages 51 to 70 (1,000 mg)
Females ages 51 to 71 (1200 mg)
Males and females age 71 and older (1,200 mg)

Please remember that this reflects your total calcium intake from food, drinks, and/or supplements. Try to avoid supplementing 100 percent of your recommended calcium intake unless directed to do so by a physician. The daily upper limit is:

2,500 mg for adults 19 to 50 years of age
2,000 mg for adults 51 years and older

If you are not being monitored by a physician, try keeping daily calcium supplementation at or below 500 mg. In addition, 90—150 mcg of vitamin K2 a few days per week in the form of MK-7 should be considered (see *Vitamin K2*).

Table 9. Calcium—Food Type and Supplement Schedule

Food Type	When	How Often
milk yogurt cheese kale broccoli canned fish with soft bones (e.g., sardines, salmon) orange juice (calcium fortified)	✓ With meals ✓ Between meals	❑ Any one of these food items 2 times a day

Or Supplement		
Calcium citrate (absorbs extremely well with food or on an empty stomach) Calcium carbonate (absorbs well with food; less expensive than calcium citrate)		

Brand	When		How Often
Citracal Petites – Calcium Citrate (200 mg each) Vitamin D3 (250 IU each)	✓ With meals ✓ Between meals ✗ NOT with zinc or iron supplement	Maintenance Phase (only)	❑ 1 or 2 pills a day This is ¼ to ½ the manufacturer's recommendation
Any reputable manufacturer	✓ As directed	Maintenance Phase (only)	Do not exceed 500 mg of supplemental calcium per day unless directed to do so by your physician.

Absorption Inhibitors

Caffeine; vitamin D deficiency; magnesium deficiency; foods with phytate, such as wheat bran, pinto beans, navy beans and peas; and foods that contain oxalates, such as beets, spinach, rhubarb, okra, tea, and sweet potatoes, inhibit calcium absorption.

Excessive protein consumption depletes calcium from your bones and may require higher calcium intake (see *Protein*).

Absorption Enhancers

Vitamin D, vitamin K2, magnesium, and lysine greatly enhance the absorption and utilization of calcium. Note, however, that calcium inhibits the absorption of magnesium.

When magnesium is included in a calcium supplement, it may enhance calcium absorption, but calcium will inhibit absorption of the included magnesium. Do not rely on calcium supplements that contain magnesium to significantly increase your magnesium levels.

Preferred Product

Citracal Petites absorb extremely with or without food. Each serving (2 pills) contains 400 mg of (elemental) calcium and 500 IU of vitamin D3. The tablets are fairly small and easy to swallow.

There are other reputable manufacturers that sell high-quality calcium supplements. Choose the one that is right for you.

Personal

I supplement with Citracal Petites at one-fourth to one-half of the recommended dosage. The product label suggests taking four pills a day to obtain 80 percent of the RDA for calcium. I alternate between taking one pill a day and two pills a day. I also consume calcium-rich foods such as milk, orange juice, and kale.

Listen to Your Body

Due to your body's tight regulation on calcium in your blood serum by releasing it from your bones, calcium deficiency can go undetected until you begin to suffer from bone-health issues.

Excess calcium may result in symptoms such as constipation or kidney stones. However, kidney stones can be caused by other issues.

Warning

There has been some discussion over a potential link between calcium supplementation and increased risk of heart disease. Lack of K2 may be a contributing factor.

Do not avoid calcium supplements. Nevertheless, consider not exceeding 500 mg of (elemental) calcium supplementation a day. Be cognizant of foods and products that inadvertently trigger the release of calcium from your bones into your bloodstream such as excessive protein. I am not suggesting protein is bad for you or that it should be avoided. I am suggesting that high protein intake should be balanced with appropriate (not excessive) magnesium, D3, calcium and K2.

If a physician recommends supplementing more than 500 mg of calcium a day, discuss any concerns you may have regarding increased risk of heart disease and the potential for impeding the absorption of other minerals in food or supplements when taken with calcium. In addition, ask your physician's views on looking at your magnesium levels (epithelial cell analysis), vitamin K2 intake (via diet history), and vitamin D levels.

Testing

Blood serum tests for calcium levels are very common. However, your body keeps tight regulation on calcium levels in your blood stream by releasing calcium from your bones when needed.

A sublingual epithelial cell analysis [2] may be considered for measuring calcium levels within your tissue. The test kit is shipped to your local physician who collects small soft-tissue samples from the mouth. Individuals who have undergone the process state that the procedure is noninvasive and virtually painless. Tissue analysis results include levels and ratios for the following elements, magnesium, phosphorous, potassium, calcium, sodium, and chloride.

You are encouraged to engage in additional research before subjecting yourself to any testing procedure. For more information, please visit www.notthecans.com/info/.

As mentioned in a previous chapter (see *Vitamin K2*), another calcium testing method worth strong consideration is the coronary calcium scan.[3] The coronary calcium scan looks for specks of calcium in the walls of the coronary (heart) arteries. Two machines can perform the scan—electron beam computed tomography (EBCT) and multidetector computed tomography (MDCT). Calcifications in the coronary arteries are an early sign of coronary heart disease (CHD).

Additional information on the coronary calcium scan is available at: http://www.nhlbi.nih.gov/health/health-topics/topics/cscan/

[1] Bunyaratavej N, Buranasinsup S. (2011 Oct) Calcium supplement: humanity's double-edged sword. Journal of the Medical Association of Thailand. 94 Suppl 5:S56-8.
[2] "Magnesium and Heart Disease", accessed August 27, 2014, http://www.exatest.com/
[3] "What Is a Coronary Calcium Scan?" accessed July 18, 2014, http://www.nhlbi.nih.gov/health/health-topics/topics/cscan/

Multivitamins and Minerals

Everything (Hair, Skin, Organ Health, Focus, Energy, Immune System, Depression, etc.)

Multivitamins/minerals (MVM) are a compilation of vitamins, minerals, and trace elements needed to sustain physical and mental well-being. The National Institutes of Health[1] states, "Women, the elderly, people with more education, more income, healthier diets and lifestyles, and lower body weights, and people in the western United States use MVMs most often. Smokers and members of certain ethnic and racial groups (such as African Americans, Hispanics, and Native Americans) are less likely to take a daily MVM."

An editorial published by the *Annals of Internal Medicine*[2] claims that vitamin and mineral supplements are a waste of money. Upon reading the article, certain statements caught my attention, such as:

> efficacy of vitamin supplements for primary prevention in community-dwelling adults <u>with no nutritional deficiencies</u>

> use of a multivitamin supplement in a <u>well-nourished elderly population</u> did not prevent cognitive decline

I agree with the conclusion that vitamin and mineral supplements may not benefit people who are "well nourished" and people "with no nutritional deficiencies." However, people who do suffer from nutrient deficiencies can benefit immensely from supplementation. I would also argue, supplements are the very reason that some people do not have nutritional deficiencies. The editorial resulted in the following headlines.

> "Experts: Don't Waste Your Money on Multivitamins" (*WebMD*)
> "Vitamins Lack Clear Health Benefits, May Pose Risks" (*Forbes*)
> "Medical journal: 'Case closed' against vitamin pills" (*USA Today*)

I am deeply concerned by the message that is being conveyed as it may persuade individuals who do have nutritional deficiencies to not consider vitamin or mineral supplements as a means to improve their health and performance. In contrast, the Harvard School of Public Health [3] states, "Looking at all the evidence, the potential health benefits of taking a standard daily multivitamin seem to outweigh the potential risks for most people."

The Agency for Healthcare Research and Quality [4] states, "Multivitamin/ mineral supplement use may prevent cancer in individuals with poor or suboptimal nutritional status."

In addition, specialized formulations of MVMs are recommended or prescribed for prenatal care. This is likely because a high-quality MVM is far more efficient at filling a broad-spectrum of nutritional gaps. They cannot and should not be used in place of healthy food choices. They most definitely should be used to "top-off" your nutritional tank when diet alone does not meet all of your requirements.

I have personally witnessed the impact of a high-quality MVM on individuals who were nutrient deficient. For example, I gave a female doctor and a homeless man a seven-day supply of MVMs each. They were both amazed by the difference they felt. The doctor had been suffering from chronic fatigue. She attributed her condition to work related stress. Within a week of taking the MVM, she was astonished by the significant improvement in her focus and energy. The homeless man had been suffering from a severe and frequent cough for more than a month. Within three days of continuous use of the MVM, he came to me extremely excited and said, "What did you give me? My cough is almost gone! I haven't felt this good in years! Thank you so much!"

How Much and How Often

Try any high-quality MVM six days per week for up to thirty days, either in half doses or at full strength. If you do not notice results, many retailers offer full refunds. A comprehensive list of 100 MVM products to choose from can be found at www.MultivitaminGuide.org.

Quite often, a high-quality MVM will discolor your urine with a very rich yellowish hue. Don't panic. This is mainly the excess B-12 flushing out of your system. If you are nutrient deficient, your energy and mental focus should noticeably increase in three days to two weeks. The more nutrient-deficient you are, the quicker and more noticeable the results should be. If you are prone to coughs, illnesses, or infections, you may realize a decrease in frequency, severity, and/or duration. There are many benefits that a high-quality MVM has to offer individuals with mild to severe nutrient deficiencies.

High-quality MVMs cost much more than more familiar brands. As with most things, you get what you pay for. I assign a four-tier categorization based on overall quality to MVMs. The fourth tier is the worst, and the first tier is the best. Each tier consists of several brands. First-tier brands sell for as much as $100 to $120 for a one-month supply. The pills are typically very small yet they practically work miracles. A full dose may require seven or more pills per day. I normally stay within the second-tier range, which costs around $18 for a one-month supply. First- and second-tier brands have an exceedingly high absorption rate. Consider taking only one-third or one-half of the recommended dose per day even if it requires you to break a pill in half. For instance, if the manufacturer's recommendation is two pills per day, break one pill in half. Take one-half with breakfast and the other half during lunch. Not only will you obtain the additional nutrients you need, but your supply will last twice as long which translates into savings. Individuals who drink alcohol excessively or maintain a very poor diet may require the full recommended dose.

First-tier MVMs normally contain a very balanced ratio of vitamins, minerals, and trace elements. Second-tier MVMs sometimes contain extreme amounts of some vitamins. Third and fourth-tier MVMs are of extremely poor-quality and may sell for as low as $20 for a one-year supply (approx. $1.67 per month). They use the least desirable forms of vitamins and minerals and are one-step removed from a placebo. They seem to put more money into TV advertisements than the vitamins themselves. In the long run, investing in a high-quality MVM may be more cost-effective due to the potential mental and physical health benefits.

Many MVMs contain poor-quality minerals such as magnesium oxide. Poor-quality minerals do not absorb well and do not provide much of your daily intake. In addition, minerals compete for the same absorption receptors, which is why some minerals strongly inhibit the absorption of other minerals.

Excess nutrients from MVMs combined with a nutrient-rich diet can introduce health problems. Individuals who regularly take MVMs typically maintain a healthier diet than those who do not. If your diet is reasonably sound, consider moderating your high-quality MVM intake by only taking half (or less) of the manufacturer's recommended serving. In addition, do not take a MVM every day. Five or six days per week should be more than sufficient. There is no benefit to overdosing nutrients. Doing so simply wastes money and it can be detrimental to your long-term health. If your diet is nutrient-poor, taking the full recommended serving, five to seven days per week may be required.

Supplements are not designed to supply all of your nutritional needs. They are merely a means to fill nutritional gaps in your diet (see *Supplement Abuse*).

Table 10. MultivaminGuide.org—Multivitamins (25 of 100) i

Company	Product
Xtend-Life Natural Products	Total Balance
Shaklee	Vitalizer Gold
Douglas Laboratories	Ultra Preventive X
USANA Health Sciences	HealthPak
Life Extension	Life Extension Mix
Metagenics	Wellness Essentials
Nutrilite (Amway, Quixtar)	Double X
Garden of Life	Vitamin Code
Source Naturals	Life Force
Karuna	Maxxum 4
Solgar	Omnium
Optimum Nutrition	Opti-Men
Muscle Pharm	Armour-V
Dr. Julian Whitaker's	Forward Multi-Nutrient
FreeLife	Reverse!
Mountain Naturals of Vermont	Superior Care
Amni	Added Protection III
Purity Products	Perfect Multi Focus Formula
Universal Nutrition	Animal Pak
Doctor's Nutrition	Mega Vites
DaVinci Laboratories	Spectra
GNC	GNC Mega Men Sport
TwinLab	Daily One Caps with Iron
FoodScience of Vermont	Superior Care
Puritan's Pride	High Potency Ultra Vita Time Release

Absorption Inhibitors

Absorption can be inhibited by phytate and caffeine.

i   Criteria used to compare multivitamin brands can be found at: http://www.multivitaminguide.org/study-methodology.html

Absorption Enhancers

Multivitamins/minerals are absorbed best when taken with a meal.

Preferred Product

Optimum Nutrition Opti-Men/Opti-Women and GNC (Mega) MVM.

Personal

I take Optimum Nutrition Opti-Men vitamins. I take one-half of a pill with breakfast. I take one whole pill with lunch. The recommend serving is three pills per day. In addition, due to a healthy diet, I skip one or two days of taking an MVM per week to diminish potential nutrient excess.

Listen to Your Body

General symptoms of a deficiency may include fatigue, insomnia, hair loss, dry skin, headache, depression, anxiety, frequent infections, and slow healing. Excess may cause stomach cramps, nausea, or diarrhea.

Warning

Multivitamins can irritate your stomach especially if not taken with a meal. Symptoms include stomach cramps, nausea, and diarrhea.

Testing

Each nutrient type contained in a MVM requires specific tests.

[1] "Multivitamin/mineral Supplements Fact Sheet for Health Professionals," last reviewed Jan 07, 2013, http://ods.od.nih.gov/factsheets/MVMS-HealthProfessional/

[2] Guallar E, Stranges S, Mulrow C, et al. (2013 Dec 17) Enough Is Enough: Stop Wasting Money on Vitamin and Mineral Supplements. *Annals of Internal Medicine.* 159(12):850-851. doi:10.7326/0003-4819-159-12-201312170-00011

[3] "A daily multivitamin is a great nutrition insurance policy," accessed July 27, 2014, http://www.hsph.harvard.edu/nutritionsource/what-should-you-eat/vitamins/

[4] Huang HY, Caballero B, Chang S, et al. (2006 May) The Efficacy and Safety of Multivitamin and Mineral Supplement Use to Prevent Cancer and Chronic Disease in Adults: A Systematic Review for a National Institutes of Health State-of-the-Science Conference. *Annals of Internal Medicine,* 145:372-385. doi:10.7326/0003-4819-145-5-200609050-00135

Protein

Immune System, Mental Health, Liver Disease, Heart Health, Bone Density, Healing, Hair Health

Proteins are one of the body's most utilized sources for building tissue and for brain function. Inadequate protein intake is extremely unhealthy and can lead to growth retardation (in children), reduction in muscle mass, decreased immunity, heart issues, and more.

Excessive protein can be unhealthy for individuals with impaired liver or kidney function. Hepatic encephalopathy is a worsening of brain function that occurs when the liver can no longer remove toxic substances in the blood.

Excessive protein, coupled with low mineral intake can lower serum pH resulting in acidosis. The body reacts to acidosis by releasing calcium from the bones to regain the proper pH balance, which can affect bone density. You can counteract some of the acidic effects of excess protein with fruits and dark green vegetables. Also, ensure you are obtaining adequate (not excessive) magnesium, potassium, calcium, and phosphorus to maintain the balance.

Please keep in mind. You do need a continuous supply of protein for optimum health. In addition, a healthy individual can process high levels of protein without any known associated risk. With animal-based proteins, closely monitor your fat and cholesterol intake. In addition, research indicates a direct correlation between heavy red meat consumption an increased risk of Cardio Vascular Disease (CVD) and cancer mortality.[1] Red meat cooking methods may also be a factor.

You will find a handy weight-based protein calculator at www.proteinsmart.kashi.com. Excessive protein intake for workout enthusiasts is not beneficial to muscle gain. In fact, it can prevent you from reaching your fitness goals. One should only consume the amount of protein required to maintain their health and reach their fitness goals. More is not better.

Avoid high intake of soy-based products. Here again, we learn years later that something promoted as being good for you significantly increases certain health risks such as breast cancer. Soy also contains high levels of phytic acid, which reduces the body's ability to absorb magnesium, zinc, calcium, iron, and other minerals. High soy intake has been shown to lower sperm concentration in men.[2]

Some of the preferred products listed in this book may contain soy as low levels are perfectly fine. Read the labels carefully.

Vegetarians

Vegetarians can get enough basic protein via plants. However, important amino acids, such as L-taurine and L-lysine, are only abundant in animal-based protein. L-lysine is one of nine essential amino acids that cannot be manufactured by your body. The good news is that L-taurine and L-lysine can be supplemented.

How Much and How Often

Protein intake for a moderately active person should fall between 0.35 g and 0.4 g of protein per pound of body weight. Advanced exercise regimens will likely require higher protein intake in the range of 0.4 to 0.6 g per pound. Professional athlete requirements may hover around 0.7 g to 0.8 g of protein per pound of body weight during training. Heavy lifting at the local gym does not require professional athlete levels of protein intake.

Beverages such as milk contain protein and carbohydrates. If using protein and carb powders with milk or juice, add the number of milligrams (mg) listed on the label with the amount contained in the powders you are adding. If your objective is to consume 25 grams of protein in one serving, a serving of milk contains 8 grams and Super Seed fiber contains 6 grams. Therefore you only need to add an additional 11 grams of protein powder to achieve 25 grams in total. This concept is also true regarding carbohydrates.

Unfortunately, at the gym I see a lot of emphasis placed on protein and amino acids, with little discussion regarding potassium, magnesium, calcium, and phosphorous. Training that requires more protein, also requires more potassium, magnesium, calcium, and phosphorous to build and maintain strong tissue. K2 is also needed to keep your arteries clear of calcium, allowing unrestricted blood flow to and from your heart.

These elements need to be kept in balance for optimum health, performance, and results at the gym. In addition, a balanced nutrient approach will provide your muscles, tendons, bones, and joints better protection against, and a speedier recovery from, injury. Adequate (not excessive) zinc intake can also play a major role in achieving optimum hysical conditioning. You are encouraged to adapt a nutrient-balance strategy to accomplish and maintain your goals.

Table 11. Protein—Food Type and Supplement Schedule

Food Type	When	How Much Per Day
tuna, chicken, turkey, bison, lean beef or pork, wild salmon, tilapia, white fish, shellfish, cage free eggs, milk, cheese (dairy), beans, seeds, nuts, nut butter	✓ With meals ✓ Between meals	0.35 to 0.5 grams for every pound of body weight. Consume 1 to 2 grams of healthy carbs for every gram of protein together or separately. Advanced exercise regimens may require higher protein intake.

Or Supplement

Whey isolate protein powder (absorbs extremely well)

Brand	When	How Often
Optimum Nutrition – Whey Protein Isolate Powder (or any reputable manufacturer)	✓ Between meals ✓ Meal replacement ✓ Add to milk, juice, water, smoothie, etc. ✓ carbohydrate powder (optional) Maintenance Phase (only)	❑ 0.1 to 0.2 grams per pound of body weight every other day or as needed ❑ 0.15 to 0.25 grams per pound of body weight for advanced exercise regimens Consume 1 to 2 grams of healthy carbs for every gram of protein. Supplemental protein should NOT provide the majority of your daily requirement.

Absorption Inhibitors

Protein absorption is rarely inhibited within a healthy GI tract.

Absorption Enhancers

Papaya, cheeses, and certain vegetables provide digestive enzymes to more effectively break down protein-rich meals.

Preferred Product

Optimum Nutrition's Whey Protein Powder contains 24 g of protein, 5.5 g of branched-chain amino acids (BCAAs), and 4 g of glutamine per serving. It is loaded with whey protein isolates, which absorb exceptionally well.

Personal

I currently consume approximately 75 g of protein per day via food, beverages, and powdered supplements (0.375 g multiplied by 200 lbs). When I exercise, my daily protein intake increases to roughly 95 g per day (0.475 g multiplied by 200 lbs).

Listen to Your Body

Symptoms of protein deficiency include; skin discoloration, skin rashes, lethargy, fatigue, difficulty sleeping, excessive sleeping (lack of energy), muscle weakness, muscle loss, frequent infections, slow wound healing, hair loss, brittle hair, mood swings, depression, anxiety, and apathy.

Excessive protein may present itself as low calcium, gout, or kidney stones.

Warning

There are some health-risks associated with excessive protein intake especially for individuals with impaired kidney or liver function. Potential risks include cancer (not caused by protein itself, may be caused by cancer promoting agents in some protein sources and by food preparation).

[1] Pan A, Sun Q, Bernstein AM, et al. (2011 April 9) Red meat consumption and mortality: results from 2 prospective cohort studies. *Archives of Internal Medicine.* 172(7):555-63. doi: 10.1001/archinternmed.2011.2287.

[2] Chavarro JE1, Toth TL, Sadio SM, et al. (2008 Nov). Soy food and isoflavone intake in relation to semen quality parameters among men from an infertility clinic. *Human Reproduction (Oxford, England).* 23(11):2584-90. doi: 10.1093/humrep/den243.

Fiber

Heart Health, Stroke, Hypertension, Diabetes, Weight Loss

In the United States, most people consume less than the required amount of fiber needed to manage weight and maintain optimum health. As stated on Medline Plus,[1] "Dietary fiber adds bulk to your diet and makes you feel full faster, helping you control your weight. It helps digestion and helps prevent constipation. Most Americans don't eat enough dietary fiber. But add it to your diet slowly. Increasing dietary fiber too quickly can lead to gas, bloating, and cramps."

There are two forms of fiber: soluble and insoluble. Soluble fiber absorbs water and forms a gel, slowing digestion. Soluble fiber is found in the following:

- Oatmeal
- Oat bran
- Nuts and seeds
- Most fruits (e.g., strawberries, blueberries, pears, and apples)
- Dry beans and peas

Insoluble fiber adds bulk to the stool and appears to help food pass more quickly. It is found in foods such as:

- Whole wheat bread
- Barley
- Brown rice
- Couscous
- Bulgur or whole grain cereals
- Wheat bran
- Seeds
- Most vegetables
- Fruits

According to a study[2] published in *Nutrition Reviews*, average fiber intakes in the United States is less than half of the recommended levels.

Another study[3] published in the journal *Nutrition* concluded that adults in the United States, on average, consume less than 50 percent of the recommended levels of fiber. The study also points out that people who follow low-carbohydrate diets consume even less. In addition, dietary fiber could play a key role in curtailing obesity within the United States and other developed countries.

Individuals seeking a flatter stomach should measure their fiber intake to see if daily requirements are met. Fiber-rich diets reduce low-density lipoprotein (LDL) cholesterol, which lowers the risk of heart attack and stroke.

Fiber acts like an adhesive scrub brush, pulling substances out of the intestines and colon. Individuals with low fiber intake create an intestinal environment conducive to parasitic growth.

How Much and How Often

There currently is no RDA for fiber. The Food and Nutrition Board, National Academies Press [4] established dietary reference intakes. The following table is based on those recommendations.

Table 12. Fiber- Adequate Intake (AI).

Infants		Females	
0–6 months old	Not determined	9–18 years old	26 grams a day
7–12 months old	Not determined	19–50 years old	25 grams a day
		≥ 50 years old	21 grams a day
Children			
1–3 years old	19 grams a day	**Pregnancy**	
4–8 years old	25 grams a day	≤ 18 years old	28 grams a day
		19-50 years old	28 grams a day
Males			
9–13 years old	31 grams a day	**Lactation**	
14–50 years old	38 grams a day	≤ 18 years old	29 grams a day
≥ 50 years old	30 grams a day	19-50 years old	29 grams a day

If you have not maintained adequate fiber intake, you may suffer slight discomfort for a few days during the initial increase. Your bacterial flora should adjust and the discomfort should subside. Within a few days, the first obvious benefit will be noticeably fuller bowel movements. You should also feel full for longer periods. If your belly is distended it may appear slightly flatter within several weeks.

You may even discover intestinal parasites. Individuals can have intestinal parasites and not be aware of it. Symptoms such as fatigue, headaches, or changes in appetite are often misinterpreted or ignored.

There are very effective over-the-counter products you can take to get rid of intestinal parasites. ParaGone is one of them. If you have the stomach for it (pun intended), it would be prudent to take a sample of the parasite to your health care provider to correctly identify the species. In addition, if you are infested, there is a strong likelihood that other residents in your household are as well.

Absorption Inhibitors

Fiber, for the most part, is not absorbed.

Absorption Enhancers

Fiber, for the most part, is not absorbed.

Preferred Product

Bob's Red Mill High-Fiber Oat Bran Cereal is a rich source of fiber. Fruits, vegetables, seeds, and nuts are as well. Garden of Life Super Seed Beyond Fiber is another product worth considering.

Personal

I enjoy adding flaxseed meal to Bob's Red Mill High-Fiber Oat Bran Cereal. Each oat bran serving contains 7 g of fiber in addition to the flaxseed. I enjoy Fiber One Original Bran Cereal which contains a whopping 14 g of fiber per serving. I also eat strawberries (alone, in smoothies, in salads), pineapple, kale, vegetables (raw and cooked), beans, and baked (or microwaved) yams. I find cinnamon and honey to be a winning combination with oats. I take supplements at least one hour before or one and a half hours after eating oats.

Warning

Drink plenty of fluids with high-fiber intake. Fiber can inhibit the absorption of certain nutrients.

[1] "Dietary Fiber", laste updated July 31, 3014, http://www.nlm.nih.gov/medlineplus/dietaryfiber.html

[2] Anderson JW, Baird P, Davis RH Jr, Ferreri S, et al. (2009 Apr). Health benefits of dietary fiber. Nutr. Rev. 67(4):188-205

[3] Slavin JL, (2005 Mar), Dietary fiber and body weight, Nutrition. 21(3):411–418 doi: http://dx.doi.org/10.1016/j.nut.2004.08.018

[4] Institute of Medicine. Dietary, Functional, and Total Fiber. Dietary Reference Intakes for Energy, Carbohydrate, Fiber, Fat, Fatty Acids, Cholesterol, Protein, and Amino Acids. (2002). Washington, D. C. National Academies Press. Summary:7-8

Other Nutrients

Vitamin C (external use)
Hair, Skin, Asthma

According to the Environmental Protection Agency (EPA),[1]

> To protect drinking water from disease-causing organisms, or pathogens, water suppliers often add a disinfectant, such as chlorine, to drinking water. However, disinfection practices can be complicated because certain microbial pathogens, such as cryptosporidium, are highly resistant to traditional disinfection practices. Also, disinfectants themselves can react with naturally-occurring materials in the water to form byproducts, such as trihalomethanes and haloacetic acids, which may pose health risks.
>
> Chloramines are most commonly formed when ammonia is added to chlorine to treat drinking water. Chloramines have been used by water utilities for almost ninety years, and their use is closely regulated.

According to a study published in the European Society for Clinical Respiratory Physiology,[2] airborne chloramines can induce asthma. Although this study refers to chloramines in the air above swimming pools, the same principles apply to all chlorine-treated water.

Chloramines cannot be removed from water by reverse osmosis[i], deionization, boiling, distilling, or standing uncovered. Chloramines can be removed via catalytic carbon filters but those are quite expensive. Chlorine and chloramines can dehydrate hair, irritate skin, and cause anemia. Airborne molecules can irritate respiratory pathways and lungs.

Three hundred mg of vitamin C (ascorbic acid) will neutralize 100 percent of chlorine and chloramines in thirty gallons of water used for bathing or shaving (10 mg of C per gallon of water). In addition, vitamin C can be added to a container of water for facial cleansing or shaving.

---

[i] If the reverse osmosis system includes dual carbon filters, extended contact with regular carbon filters can neutralize chloramines in water.

A chlorine shower filter should also be considered to reduce skin and lung irritation. Due to the limited contact time with flowing water, chlorine filters do not remove chloramines, but they do remove a sizeable percentage of skin and bronchial irritants. Water testing kits are available online and at your local pet store.

CoQ10 (Coenzyme Q10)
Congestive Heart Failure (CHF), Blood Pressure, Fatigue, Depression, Gum Disease

CoQ10 is contained throughout the body. It is mostly concentrated in the liver, kidneys, heart, and pancreas. Supplemental CoQ10 has the potential for preventing cardiovascular disease.[3] Individuals who suffer from depression may also benefit from CoQ10 supplementation.[4]

People over forty years of age do not absorb CoQ10 well. Ubiquinol, a better-absorbed component of CoQ10, became available to consumers around 2006. Several years later, enhanced absorption CoQ10 was introduced, which absorbs as readily as ubiquinol and is less expensive. CoQ10 is fat-soluble and should be taken with a meal containing healthy fat. Currently, no RDA has been established for CoQ10. Research suggests 100 mg per day should be sufficient.

Carbohydrates
Energy, Weight Loss, Bone Health, Heart Health, Brain Health

Healthy carbohydrates are the body's best sources of fuel for physical endurance, brain activity, and building muscle. Not all carbs are created equal. Carbohydrates derived from bananas, berries, beans, chickpeas, yams, wild rice, and organic milk have a much healthier impact than those from cookies, doughnuts, potato chips, and soda.

Healthy carbohydrates provide several much-needed nutrients and a more stable release of glucose for adenosine triphosphate (ATP) energy. In addition, some forms of healthy carbs are high in fiber. Individuals with high intakes of dietary fiber are at significantly lower risk for developing coronary heart disease, stroke, diabetes, obesity, hypertension, and other diseases. A moderately active person should eat 0.7–1.0 g of healthy carbohydrates per pound of bodyweight. Contrary to misinformation from faux diets, healthy carbohydrates can be very beneficial to weight management and brain energy.

Studies[5] demonstrate reduced fatigue and improved exercise performance with multiple transportable carbohydrates compared with a single carbohydrate. Carbohydrate-rich foods (not processed) provide a readily available source of fuel for muscle glycogen synthesis and should be the major carbohydrate choices in workout recovery meals.

Excessive carbohydrates can be detrimental to your health. One should avoid excessive carbohydrate intake and simple carbs such as soda, sugar cookies, etc. Healthy carbohydrates in moderation are very beneficial. Nutrition is comprehensive, not binary (all or nothing).

Essential Fatty Acids—Omega 3
Heart Health, Brain Health, Weight Loss

According to the Office of Dietary Supplements,[6] there are two major classes of polyunsaturated fatty acids, omega-3 (alpha-linolenic acid, or ALA) and omega-6 (linoleic acid, or LA). Omega-3 and omega-6 fatty acids cannot be made by the body and therefore must be obtained through food, beverages, or supplements.

Most Americans consume more than ten times more omega-6 (LA) than omega-3 (ALA), which means the ratio of omega-6 to omega-3 consumption is more than 10:1. The ratio for good health, however, should be roughly 3:1. To achieve this balance, individuals should consume more omega-3 and less omega-6 fatty acids.

Men consume significantly less omega-3 than women do. In addition, individuals with a history of cardiovascular disease (CVD) consume less omega-3 than those without CVD.

Once absorbed, omega-3 is converted to eicosapentaenoic acid (EPA) and docosahexaenoic acid (DHA) and put to use. EPA and DHA also occur naturally in some foods such as cold-water fish. Omega-3 is present in leafy green vegetables (e.g., spinach, kale), nuts, vegetable oils, and especially in flaxseed and flaxseed oil. Good sources of EPA and DHA are fish (both finfish and shellfish and their oils and eggs) and organ meats. Omega-6 is found in many foods consumed by Americans, including meat, vegetable oils (e.g., safflower, sunflower, corn, soy), and processed foods made with these oils.

Supplemental flaxseed oil provides omega-3. Fish oil provides EPA and DHA (which is also made from omega-3 inside your body). Algal oils provide a vegetarian source of DHA. Flaxseed meal provides omega-3 and a healthy dose of fiber. It can be added to a variety of dishes, salads, smoothies, and protein shakes.

High supplemental fish oil levels measured in blood have been linked to a significantly higher risk for prostate cancer.[7]

Sleep (technically not a nutrient)
Energy, Weight Loss, Bone Health, Heart Health, Brain Health, more...

According to the CDC:[8]

> Insufficient sleep is associated with a number of chronic diseases and conditions—such as diabetes, cardiovascular disease, obesity, and depression—which threaten our nation's health. Notably, insufficient sleep is associated with the onset of these diseases and also poses important implications for their management and outcome.

7 to 7.5 hours of undisturbed appears to be the healthiest duration of sleep for many adults. Sleep studies[9] have identified a possible correlation between increased incidence of natural death and:

- sleep intervals less than 6.5 hours
- sleep intervals greater than 8 hours

Preferred Products

- ✓ NutriBiotic Ascorbic Acid – Pure Vitamin C Crystalline Powder
- ✓ Sprite High Output Shower Filter
- ✓ Aquasana Shower Filter
- ✓ Jarrow Formulas Q-absorb CoQ10 (enhanced absorption)
- ✓ Bob's Red Mill Flaxseed Meal (rich in omega-3 and fiber)
- ✓ Renew Life Norwegian Critical Omega Fish Gels[i]

---

[i] Fish oil has been linked to a 44 percent higher risk for prostate cancer. Men should consider moderating intake to only three or four nonconsecutive days per week. Refer to -*Nutrients That May Prevent Prostate Cancer*- for references and additional details.

1   "Basic Information about Disinfectants in Drinking Water", accessed Dec 13, 2013, http://water.epa.gov/drink/contaminants/basicinformation/disinfectants.cfm

2   Thickett KM1, McCoach JS, Gerber JM., et al. (2002 May). Occupational asthma caused by chloramines in indoor swimming-pool air. *European Society for Clinical Respiratory Physiology, European Respiratory Journal.* 19(5):827–32.

3   Langsjoen PH, Langsjoen AM. (1999). Overview of the use of CoQ10 in cardiovascular disease. *US BioFactors.* 9(2–4):273–84

4   Maes M, Mihaylova I, Kubera M, et al. (2009). Lower plasma Coenzyme Q10 in depression. *Neuro Endocrinology Letters.* 30(4):462-9.

5   Jeukendrup AE. (2010 Jul). Carbohydrate and exercise performance: the role of multiple transportable carbohydrates. *Current Opinion in Clinical Nutrition and Metabolic Care.* 13(4):452-7. doi: 10.1097/MCO.0b013e328339de9f

6   "Omega-3 Fatty Acids and Health", last reviewed October 28, 2005, http://ods.od.nih.gov/factsheets/Omega3FattyAcidsandHealth-HealthProfessional/

7   "Fish Oil Linked to Prostate Cancer Risk", September 3, 2013, http://www.nlm.nih.gov/medlineplus/podcast/transcript090313.html

8   CDC. (2013 Jul 1). Sleep and Sleep Disorders. CDC, National Center for Chronic Disease Prevention and Health Promotion, Division of Population Health. http://www.cdc.gov/sleep/

9   Hublin C, Partinen M, Koskenvuo M, et al. (2007). Sleep and mortality: a population-based 22-year follow-up study. *Sleep.* 30(10):1245-1253.

Nutrient-Based Remedies
(Consult with a Physician)

Insomnia

- Taurine: supplement 500–1000 mg, four to six nights per week with dinner or late night snack (see *Taurine*)
- Magnesium: supplement 100–200 mg one hour before bed and an additional 100 mg to 200 mg just before bed (do not count magnesium oxide) (see *Magnesium*)
- Potassium: consume potassium-rich foods, low-sodium V8, and coconut water and/or supplement 400–800 mg in divided doses each day with meals (see *Potassium*)
- Vitamin C: reduce your vitamin C intake if you are taking more than 250 mg per day; avoid vitamin C-rich foods within three hours prior to sleeping
- High-quality Chamomile Tea (mild to moderate insomnia) or Yogi Bedtime Tea (severe insomnia): 30 minutes before bed
- Vitamin K2 as MK7: supplement 100 mcg, three to five days per week. (see *Vitamin K2*)
- Vitamin D: 8,400–14,000 mg per week via food, beverages, or supplements (*see Vitamin D3*)
- Sleep: It appears that 7–7 ½ hours of undisturbed sleep is the healthiest duration of sleep for most adults. Human beings are unique so there will always be exceptions

Fatigue

- Multivitamin: high quality (*see Multivitamins and Minerals*)
- Vitamin B12: can be obtained from a multivitamin
- Iron: 18–25 mg, two to three days per week (*see Iron*)
- Zinc: 15–25 mg, three to four days per week (see Zinc)
- Magnesium: 200–400 mg before bed (*see Magnesium*)
- Potassium: consume potassium-rich foods, low-sodium v8, and coconut water and/or supplement 400–800 mg in divided doses each day with meals (*see Potassium*)
- Healthy carbohydrates: 0.5–0.75 g per pound of body weight (*see Other Nutrients*)

- Protein: 0.35–0.5 g per pound of bodyweight (*see Protein*)
- ParaGone (optional): intestinal parasites can cause fatigue
- Seven to 7 ½ hours of undisturbed sleep (refer to *Insomnia*)

Low Testosterone

- Zinc: 15–25 mg, three to four days per week (see Zinc)
- Cage-free eggs: 1 egg three to five days per week (testosterone is made from cholesterol)
- Iodine: 50–100 mcg three to five days per week, or 300–500 mcg one or two days per week
- Iron: supplement 18–25 mg, one to three days per week (*see Iron*)
- Seven to 7 ½ hours of undisturbed sleep (refer to Insomnia)

Cold Sores
Prevent Cold Sore Formation and Accelerate Healing

- Quantum's Super Lysine Plus: as directed at first sign of an outbreak such as tingling sensation or itch. Works almost immediately (take only when needed)
- Zinc: 15–25 mg, three to four days per week (see Zinc)
- Arginine: reduce intake of arginine-rich foods, such as nuts and chocolate
- Seven to 7 ½ hours of undisturbed sleep (refer to *Insomnia*)

Asthma
Reduce Intensity and Frequency of Asthmatic Episodes

- Magnesium: 200–400 mg per day (*see Magnesium*)
- Potassium: consume potassium-rich foods, low-sodium V8, and coconut water and/or supplement 400–800 mg in divided doses each day with meals (*see Potassium*)
- Zinc: 15–25 mg, three to four days per week (see Zinc)
- Taurine: 500–1000 mg, four to six days per week with meals (*see Taurine*)
- Shower Filter: removes chlorine from water (does not remove chloramines)
- Vitamin C: add 200–300 mg to bath water to neutralize chlorine and chloramines, which can irritate air passageways when inhaled (*see Other Nutrients*)

- Omega-3: daily from food sources (salmon, flaxseed, etc.) and/or supplements (appears to reduce inflammation) (*see Other Nutrients*)
- Seven to 7 ½ hours of undisturbed sleep (refer to *Insomnia*)

Hair Loss Prevention

Hair's major components consist of the follicle, bulb, root, and shaft. The hair shaft is over 90 percent protein. Hair health is directly affected by nutrition and the health of the scalp. Many hair products focus on the shaft, yet the root and the scalp often go unattended (out of sight, out of mind). To maintain a healthy shaft, root, and scalp one should consider the following:

- Chlorine shower filter: removes chlorine from water for less scalp irritation. Does not remove chloramines
- Omega-3: daily from food sources (salmon, flaxseed, etc.) and/or supplements
- Protein: for hair growth and strength (*see Protein*)
- Zinc: 15–25 mg, three to four days per week (see Zinc)
- Iodine: 50–100 mcg two to four nonconsecutive days per week, or 300–500 mcg one or two nonconsecutive days per week (see *Iodine*)
- Iron: from food, or supplement 18–25 mg, two to three days per week (*see Iron*)
- Multivitamin: high-quality (*see Multivitamins and Minerals*)
- Biotin (stand-alone supplement): 300 mcg, four to six days per week in addition to biotin in a multivitamin (excessive biotin levels can cause cystic acne and skin discoloration)
- Vitamin C: 100–250 mg per day via vitamins, food, or beverages. Excessive doses can cause oxalate kidney stones or exacerbate iron overload in people with hemochromatosis
- Vitamin D: 8,400–14,000 mg per week via food, beverages, or supplements (*see Vitamin D3*)
- Maple Holistics Hydrate Shampoo (for dry hair and flaking scalp)
- Reduce frequency and intensity of exposure to hot combs, curling irons, harsh chemicals, etc.
- Do not wash hair daily, as it dries the scalp and depletes oils. Rinse instead (use filtered water)
- UV protection: shade, UV hairspray or leave-in conditioner
- Hair moisturizer: hair is brittle when very dry (or wet)
- Pure emu (or other quality) oil: gently massage into scalp two to four days per week

- Manage stress: twenty minutes of exercise and/or twenty minutes of complete calm per day
- Seven to 7 ½ hours of undisturbed sleep (refer to *Insomnia*)

Itchy Scalp

- Chlorine shower filter: removes chlorine from water for less scalp irritation. Does not remove chloramines
- Sulfate-free shampoo
- Zinc: 15–25 mg, three to four days per week (see Zinc)
- Nizoral shampoo: use as directed for up to eight weeks. If itch stops before eight weeks, continue use for two additional weeks (contains 1 percent Ketoconazole, which is an azole antifungal. Some people may be allergic). Itching should slightly decrease after the first week and noticeably decrease after the third week. Use only as diected
- Ensure the detergent you use on your bedding does not irritate your scalp

Brittle or Cavity-Prone Teeth

- Vitamin K2 (MK7): 100–250 mcg three to six days per week (*see Vitamin K2*)
- Magnesium: 200–400 mg three to six days per week (see Magnesium)
- Vitamin D: 8,400–14,000 mg per week via food, beverages, or supplements (*see Vitamin D3*)
- Calcium: 200–500 mg four to six days per week in addition to calcium-rich foods and beverages (*see Calcium*)
- Vitamin C: 100–250 mg per day via food, beverages, or supplements
- Zinc: 18–25 mg three or four days per week (see Zinc)
- Xylitol Gum or Mints: 3–6 g per day divided into two or more doses after a snack or meal (reduces cavity causing bacteria). Do not exceed 20 g in a single day. Very toxic to dogs! Xylitol triggers a potent, life-threatening insulin release in dogs
- Water: rinse mouth after consuming acidic meals or beverages
- Now solutions Xyli-White toothpaste (fluoride-free)
- Rinse mouth with water following consuming acidic foods
- Remineralizing toothpaste, rinses, or gels
- Phosphorus deficiency can result in sudden tooth decay. Excessive phosphorus can be hazardous to your health

Muscle Cramps, Pulls, and Knots

- Magnesium: 200–400 mg per day (*see Magnesium*)
- Potassium: consume potassium-rich foods, low-sodium V8, and coconut water and/or supplement 400–800 mg in divided doses each day with meals (*see Potassium*)
- Taurine: 500–1,000 mg, four to six days per week (*see Taurine*)
- Vitamin D: 8,400–14,000 IU per week (*see Vitamin D3*)
- Water: dehydration can cause muscle cramps

Immune System
Prevent Viral Infections such as Colds and Influenza (flu). Improve Wound Healing

- Zinc: 18–25 mg three or four days per week (see Zinc)
- Vitamin D: 8,400–14,000 IU per week (*see Vitamin D3*)
- Vitamin C: 100–250 mg per day via food, beverages, or supplements.
- Multivitamin: high-quality (*see Multivitamins and Minerals*)
- Seven to 7 ½ hours of undisturbed sleep (refer to *Insomnia*)

Razor Bumps
Lessen Severity

- Vitamin C (external): neutralizes 100 percent of chlorine and chloramines in water reducing dryness and irritation. Add 200–300 mg to bath for bathing or shaving. Add 20–30 mg to a large bowl of water for facial cleansing and shaving. Use a cup to scoop water out of the bowl. Rinse razors and skin with treated water over a drain (see *Other Nutrients*)
- Chlorine shower filter: removes chlorine from water, which reduces skin irritation (*see Other Nutrients*)
- Pre-shave Oil: Pre-shave oils do a remarkable job at reducing skin irritation during shaving. You can purchase a pre-shave oil or even make it yourself. A recipe published by Donna Tinus on eHow.com[i] states: Pour 1 cup Castor oil, 1/2 cup olive oil and 5 drops of sandalwood essential oil into a tinted glass or plastic container with a lid. Shake the container well to mix the ingredient

---

[i] Pre-shave oil recipe provided by Donna Tinus. Originally published on eHow.com. ©Demand Media, Inc. All rights reserved.

Supplement Abuse

You have just finished reading about a variety of nutrients that can improve your health and overall quality of life. With this in mind, I strongly encourage you to avoid the growing wave of supplement abuse.

A ten year study published in *Hepatology* (2014) shows liver injury caused by herbals and dietary supplements (HDS) has increased from seven percent to 20 percent.

Megadosing and Overuse of Supplements

A ten year study [1] published in *Hepatology* (2014) shows liver injury caused by herbals and dietary supplements (HDS) has increased from seven percent to 20 percent

According to *Merriam-Webster*,[2] a supplement is "something that is added to something else in order to make it complete." Unfortunately, some people have convinced themselves and others that their bodies function better with excessive doses of nutrients instead of a balanced ratio. Hospitalizations and premature deaths caused by long-term, excessive supplementation are likely misdiagnosed or written off as natural causes. Hospital questionnaires are not very probative regarding type of supplements and dosage a patient regularly consumes.

Vitamin E is a good example of a potential silent killer at high doses. A meta-analysis published in 2005 [3] indicates that regular vitamin E doses of 400-IU or more may increase all-cause mortality.

The Fred Hutchinson Cancer Research Center [4] found that supplementation with vitamin E resulted in a 63 percent increased risk for prostate cancer and a 111 percent increased risk for high-grade cancer status among men with low selenium. High doses of vitamin E can also result in excessive bleeding when injured.

In addition, high levels of fish oil intake have been linked to a 44 percent higher risk for developing prostate cancer.[5]

It would be a disservice to exclude a study [6] that concluded that 600 IU of natural-source vitamin E taken every other day (300 IU daily average) decreased cardiovascular mortality in healthy women. I am not an advocate against supplements. I am an advocate against taking excessive amounts of supplements in pursuit of short-term benefits.

Iodine supplement abuse appears to be on the rise. Although the RDA for iodine is only 150 mcg per day, individuals are suggesting daily supplementation as high as 12.5 mg a day. This is more than 83 times the RDA. As stated in an earlier chapter, the belief that people in Japan consume 13.8 mg of iodine a day may have resulted from an incorrectly applied equation used on a research paper written in 1967 (*see Iodine*).

As of 2004, average iodine intakes in the United States ranged from 138 mcg to 353 mcg per day.[7] Based on actual intake levels, if 12.5 mg of daily iodine were required to maintain thyroid health, one would expect the majority of the population to develop goiter and other dramatic health issues associated with severe iodine deficiency. In addition, early stage brain development in the majority of newborns would be severely impaired. To imply that people are severely iodine deficient (compared to actual daily intake) without displaying known, associated symptoms is very problematic and extremely misleading. If individuals who encourage megadosing on iodine (or any supplement) reject the science, I urge them to consider the logic.

In addition, how much you consume of any vitamin or mineral is not nearly as important as how much you actually absorb. For instance, your body will absorb far more magnesium from 400 mg of chelated, magnesium glycinate than it will from 1000 mg of magnesium oxide. Mega-dosers often fail to differentiate between formulations that barely absorb into your system and those that are absorbed extremely well.

Also, individuals who megadose without medical supervision:

1. may not have their kidneys or liver periodically tested for stress or damage
2. may not have vitamin and mineral levels periodically checked to ensure they have not exceeded the range of safety
3. likely megadose on multiple supplements
4. may not be aware that nutrients create waste when they are broken down into components that cells can use
5. rarely differentiate between forms of nutrients that absorb extremely well and forms that do not. Highly absorbable forms of nutrients can easily exceed safe levels over time
6. may base their decision to megadose on one-off studies, speculation, misinformation, or blogger hype
7. may not be aware that articles that support megadosing on a specific supplement, such as iodine, often rely on very few sources versus multiple, credible, independent studies

8. ignore the compilation of scientific studies conducted in multiple countries that draw similar conclusions
9. may megadose on one nutrient to counteract health issues that were the result of megadosing on another nutrient
10. fail to consider the amount of nutrients naturally obtained from food and beverages

Replacing Your Body's Natural Processes

Examples of supplements some have used to replace their bodies' natural functions are digestive enzymes, and colon cleansers.

There are valid medical reasons for some people to take supplements on a frequent basis. Over the years, perfectly healthy individuals have convinced themselves and others that their bodies cannot perform some natural functions without the aid of a pill or powder.

For example, the average person does not need to ingest digestive enzymes on a daily basis. Your body can indeed digest food without the aid of a pill. Any healthy person who ingests digestive enzymes on a daily basis—or, worse, with every meal—is abusing the supplement.

Use of digestive enzymes every now and then is perfectly fine. If you are popping enzymes with every meal, you are doing your body and your wallet a disservice. You should wean yourself off by reducing the amount and frequency of consumption a little more each day. In addition, add naturally occurring digestive enzymes to your diet, such as papaya, pineapple, and green, leafy vegetables. Foods containing digestive enzymes also contain valuable nutrients and fiber; many supplemental enzymes do not.

Use of bulk forming laxatives to "cleanse the colon" and "DIY enemas" may also be occurring too frequently. Eating a healthy, fiber-filled, rounded diet is much more effective and far less harmful. Your colon contains a bacterial ecosystem that breaks down and absorbs what you need while disposing of the rest. Frequent use of harsh "natural" products disrupts this balance. Anyone without an underlying medical condition who feels the need to frequently cleanse his or her colon should reevaluate his or her diet and nutrient intake. I suspect the person has disrupted the GI tract and bacterial ecosystem via a poorly balanced diet and/or overuse of so-called healthy herbs, teas, digestive enzymes, potions, etc. Daily intake of mixed fruits, vegetables, leafy salads, cheeses, yogurt, and a little lemon juice for a few weeks may get your ecosystem back on track.

Going overboard with any substance may require going overboard with other substances to offset issues introduced by the first substance. This creates a vicious cycle that results in both psychological and physical dependency for the sake of feeling "normal." If you do not have an underlying medical condition, avoid making your body reliant on pills, herbs, or powders just to perform natural functions. Individuals with underlying health conditions are the exception.

Balance Works Better

When used properly, supplements can be very effective at maintaining one's health and performance. In general, people who take supplements make healthier food choices. Hence, individuals with healthier diets require lower doses of supplemental nutrients than those who maintain a less healthy diet. Megadosing on supplements can undermine one's investment in healthy lifestyle choices.

Your body is an extremely complex biological machine. Nutrients are like the fuel/air/spark mixture in your car's engine. Too much or too little of either one will make your engine run poorly, create more toxins, produce less energy, and shorten its life. Your cells require the right amount of air, fluids, vitamins, and minerals to operate at their peak. Overwhelming them with supplements may give you a short-term boost. Unfortunately, it may also diminish other vital functions and even shorten your life.

Always take into account that a percentage of the nutrients your body needs for optimum performance is contained in the foods you eat. As long as you stay within a certain range, your body will use or store what it needs and eliminate the rest. When you continually exceed that range, too much can be just as damaging to your health as too little.

[1]   Navarro, V. J., Barnhart, H., Bonkovsky, H. L., et al. (2014). Liver injury from herbals and dietary supplements in the U.S. Drug-Induced Liver Injury Network. *Hepatology*. doi: 10.1002/hep.27317

[2]   "Supplement", accessed Jul 25, 2014, http://www.merriam-webster.com/dictionary/supplement

[3]   Miller ER 3rd, Pastor-Barriuso R, Dalal D, Riemersma RA, et al. (2005 Jan 4). Meta-analysis: high-dosage vitamin E supplementation may increase all-cause mortality. *Annals of Internal Medicine*. 142(1):37-46.

[4]   "Selenium and vitamin E supplements can increase risk of prostate cancer in some men," Feb. 21, 2014, http://www.fhcrc.org/en/news/releases/2014/02/selenium-and-vitamin-e-supplements-can-increase-risk-of-prostate-cancer-in-some-men.html

[5]   "Fish Oil Linked to Prostate Cancer Risk", September 3, 2013, http://www.nlm.nih.gov/medlineplus/podcast/transcript090313.html

[6]   Lee IM, Cook NR, Gaziano JM, et al. (2005 Jul 6). Vitamin E in the primary prevention of cardiovascular disease and cancer: the Women's Health Study. JAMA: *American Medical Association*. 294(1):56-65.

[7]   9.Murray CW, Egan SK, Kim H, et al. (2008 Nov) US Food and Drug Administration's Total Diet Study: dietary intake of perchlorate and iodine. *J Expo Sci Environ Epidemiol*. 18(6):571-580. doi: 10.1038/sj.jes.7500648

Tainted Supplements

The Center for Drug Evaluation and Research (CDER)

According to its website, the Food and Drug Administration's (FDA) Center for Drug Evaluation and Research (CDER) promotes and protects the health of Americans by ensuring that all prescription and over-the-counter drugs are safe and effective. CDER evaluates all new drugs before they are sold, and serves as a consumer watchdog for the more than 10,000 drugs on the market to be sure they continue to meet the highest standards. The center routinely monitors TV, radio, and print drug ads to ensure they are truthful and balanced. CDER also plays a critical role in providing health professionals and consumers information to use drugs appropriately and safely.

CDER Tainted Supplement Database

On July 25, 2014, I visited the CDER Tainted Supplement webpage and found 553 tainted products listed.

Please visit CDER for a current list of tainted supplements at:
http://www.accessdata.fda.gov/scripts/sda/sdNavigation.cfm?filter=
&sortColumn=3a&sd=tainted_supplements_cder&displayAll=true

According to CDER, the list of 553 tainted products contains only a fraction of the potentially hazardous products with hidden ingredients marketed to consumers on the Internet and in retail establishments. The FDA is unable to test and identify all products marketed as dietary supplements on the market that have potentially harmful hidden ingredients. Even if a product is not included in this list, consumers should exercise caution before using certain products.

A link to the CDER Tainted Supplement Database (listed above) is also available at www.notthecans.com/info/.

Is it Really Toxic?

Virtually everything we ingest has the potential of becoming toxic (poisonous) including vitamins and minerals. The caveat to that is "at certain levels". Any substance taken in excess of what your body can safely absorb or expel can be toxic to your system. Some substances require higher amounts and longer exposure to pose a health risk.

In addition, tolerance levels are unique to each individual. For instance, gluten, for a very small percentage of people, can be a matter of life or death. Another percentage of people may have a mild, adverse reaction to it. However, moderate intake of food products that contain gluten has not been shown to pose any significant health risk to the vast majority of the population. It is possible for excessive intake of any food group, to include those containing gluten, to impose health risks. It is also possible, that today's society is engaged in a gluten-rich diet. This can be resolved by simply diversifying one's diet. Until additional, credible data becomes available, you may consider moderating your intake of gluten-based produce. With that said, do not spend much time in the gluten-free aisle. In addition, some substances used to replace gluten may be just as hazardous to your health as gluten itself.

As referenced in a previous chapter, daily intake of 400 IU (or more) of vitamin E has been shown to increase overall mortality rates. It has also been shown to significantly increase rates for developing prostate cancer as well as excessive bleeding. Yet vitamin E has not been labeled as being toxic. I am not suggesting that vitamin E is toxic and should be avoided. I do propose, however, that individuals consider moderating their vitamin E supplementation to below 400 IU per day.

For something to be toxic, we must always consider the amount, frequency, or duration of exposure it takes for a substance to pose a threat to one's health. Simply blogging that something is toxic does not relay enough information for an informed decision. Again, ingesting anything in excess of what your body can safely tolerate can be toxic to your system. Taking extreme measures due to unproven assertions, misinformation and half-truths, however, places you at greater risk for developing nutrient deficiencies and long-term health issues.

If the potential toxicity of a substance concerns you, check the facts through credible sources, such as Pubmed.gov, WebMD.com and similar sites. Bloggers and dietary-fad promoters are the least reliable sources for the information that you need to make an informed decision.

Daily Supplement Schedules

Table 13. Daily Supplement Schedule—Maintenance Phase. Ages 19–29

	Sunday	Monday	Tuesday	Wednesday	Thursday	Friday	Saturday
First Thing		300 mcg biotin		300 mcg biotin		300 mcg biotin	≤400 mg nascent iodine (optional)
Breakfast	multivitamin#, potassium*	multivitamin#, potassium*, 3000—5000 IU D3	multivitamin#, potassium*	multivitamin#, potassium*	multivitamin#, potassium*, 3000—5000 IU D3	multivitamin#, potassium*	multivitamin#, potassium*
Day & Night	fiber	fiber	fiber	fiber	fiber	fiber	fiber
Lunch		100 mcg k2 ≤22 mg zinc		100 mcg k2 ≤22 mg zinc	18 mg iron‡	100 mcg k2, ≤22 mg zinc	
Between meals	potassium*	potassium*, 200—500 mg calcium citrate	potassium*	potassium*	potassium*	potassium*, 200—500 mg calcium citrate	potassium*
Dinner	potassium*	potassium*	potassium*	potassium*	potassium*	potassium*	

90

Table 13. Daily Supplement Schedule—Maintenance Phase. Ages 19–29 (cont'd)

	Sunday	Monday	Tuesday	Wednesday	Thursday	Friday	Saturday
Day or Night		protein powder, carb powder		protein powder, carb powder		protein powder, carb powder	
Before bed	100–200 mg magnesium	100–200 mg magnesium	100–200 mg magnesium	100–200 mg magnesium	100–200 mg magnesium	100–200 mg magnesium	

* Potassium supplements (pill, powder) should always be taken with a meal. Potassium-rich foods or beverages (low-sodium V8, coconut water, banana, etc.) can be consumed with or without meals.

‡ Excess iron is extremely dangerous as it can damage your liver. For women, 18–25 mg is a moderate dose, but it should not be taken every day. Men require less iron than women. Some multivitamins contain iron, which may negate the need for additional supplementation. Please have your iron levels tested to determine how much supplementation may be right for you (if any). Please consult with a physician when considering sustained iron supplementation.

High-quality multivitamins contain high concentrations of nutrients that are absorbed extremely well. I frequently recommend not exceeding half of the manufacturer's suggested daily dose, even if that requires breaking the pill in half. I also encourage skipping one or two days per week to allow excess nutrients to be purged from your system.

Table 14. Daily Supplement Schedule—Maintenance Phase. Ages 30–39

	Sunday	Monday	Tuesday	Wednesday	Thursday	Friday	Saturday
First Thing		300 mcg biotin		300 mcg biotin		300 mcg biotin	≤400 mg nascent iodine (optional)
Breakfast	multivitamin#, potassium*	multivitamin#, potassium*, 100 mg CoQ10	multivitamin#, potassium*	multivitamin#, potassium*, 100 mg CoQ10	multivitamin#, potassium*	multivitamin#, potassium*, 100 mg CoQ10	potassium*
Day & Night	fiber	fiber	fiber	fiber	fiber	fiber	fiber
Lunch		multivitamin#, 100 mcg k2, ≤22 mg zinc, 2000 IU D3	multivitamin#, 100 mcg k2	multivitamin#, ≤22 mg zinc, 2000 IU D3	multivitamin#, 100 mcg k2, 18 mg iron‡	multivitamin#, 100 mcg k2, ≤22 mg zinc, 2000 IU D3	
Between meals	potassium*	potassium*, 200—500 mg calcium citrate	potassium*	potassium*, 200—500 mg calcium citrate	potassium*	potassium*, 200—500 mg calcium citrate	potassium*
Dinner	potassium*	potassium*	potassium*	potassium*	potassium*	potassium*	

Table 14. Daily Supplement Schedule—Maintenance Phase. Ages 30–39 (cont'd)

	Sunday	Monday	Tuesday	Wednesday	Thursday	Friday	Saturday
Day or Night		protein powder, carb powder		protein powder, carb powder		protein powder, carb powder	
Before bed	200—250 mg magnesium, 500 mg taurine	200—250 mg magnesium, 500 mg taurine	200—250 mg magnesium, 500 mg taurine	200—250 mg magnesium, 500 mg taurine	200—250 mg magnesium, 500 mg taurine	200—250 mg magnesium	

* Potassium supplements (pill, powder) should always be taken with a meal. Potassium-rich foods or beverages (low-sodium V8, coconut water, banana, etc.) can be consumed with or without meals.

‡ Excess iron is extremely dangerous as it can damage your liver. For women, 18–25 mg is a moderate dose, but it should not be taken every day. Men require less iron than women. Some multivitamins contain iron, which may negate the need for additional supplementation. Please have your iron levels tested to determine how much supplementation may be right for you (if any). Please consult with a physician when considering sustained iron supplementation.

High-quality multivitamins contain high concentrations of nutrients that are absorbed extremely well. I frequently recommend not exceeding half of the manufacturer's suggested daily dose, even if that requires breaking the pill in half. I also encourage skipping one or two days per week to allow excess nutrients to be purged from your system.

Table 15. Daily Supplement Schedule—Maintenance Phase. Ages 40+

	Sunday	Monday	Tuesday	Wednesday	Thursday	Friday	Saturday
First Thing		300 mcg biotin	300 mcg biotin	300 mcg biotin	300 mcg biotin	300 mcg biotin	≤400 mg nascent iodine (optional)
Breakfast	potassium*	multivitamin#, potassium*, 100 mg CoQ10	multivitamin#, potassium*, 100 mg CoQ10	multivitamin#, Potassium*	multivitamin#, potassium*, 100 mg CoQ10	multivitamin#, potassium*, 100 mg CoQ10	potassium*
Day & Night	fiber	fiber	fiber	fiber	fiber	fiber	fiber
Lunch	100 mcg K2, 18 mg iron‡	Multivitamin#, 100 mcg K2, ≤22 mg zinc, 2000 IU D3	multivitamin#, 100 mcg K2, ≤22 mg zinc	multivitamin#, 100 mcg K2, 18 mg iron‡, 2000 IU D3	multivitamin#, 100 mcg K2, ≤22 mg zinc	multivitamin#, 100 mcg K2, ≤22 mg zinc, 2000 IU D3	
Between meals	potassium*	potassium*, 200—500 mg calcium citrate	potassium*, 200—500 mg calcium citrate	potassium*, 200—500 mg calcium citrate	potassium*, 200—500 mg calcium citrate	potassium*, 200—500 mg calcium citrate	potassium*
Dinner	potassium*	potassium*	potassium*	potassium*	potassium*	potassium*	

Table 15. Daily Supplement Schedule—Maintenance Phase. Ages 40+ (cont'd)

Day or Night	Sunday	Monday	Tuesday	Wednesday	Thursday	Friday	Saturday
Before bed	200–400 mg magnesium, 500 mg taurine	200–400 mg magnesium, 500 mg taurine	200–400 mg magnesium, 500 mg taurine	200–400 mg magnesium, 500 mg taurine	200–400 mg magnesium, 500 mg taurine	200–400 mg magnesium	200–400 mg magnesium
		protein powder, carb powder		protein powder, carb powder		protein powder, carb powder	

* Potassium supplements (pill, powder) should always be taken with a meal. Potassium-rich foods or beverages (low-sodium V8, coconut water, banana, etc.) can be consumed with or without meals.

‡ Excess iron is extremely dangerous as it can damage your liver. For women, 18–25 mg is a moderate dose, but it should not be taken every day. Men require less iron than women. Some multivitamins contain iron, which may negate the need for additional supplementation. Please have your iron levels tested to determine how much supplementation may be right for you (if any). Please consult with a physician when considering sustained iron supplementation.

High-quality multivitamins contain high concentrations of nutrients that are absorbed extremely well. I frequently recommend not exceeding half of the manufacturer's suggested daily dose, even if that requires breaking the pill in half. I also encourage skipping one or two days per week to allow excess nutrients to be purged from your system.

Table 16. Supplements and Amounts (for Consideration)

Supplement	Amount	When	Benefits
Nutrigold—Vitamin K2 MK-7 (100 mcg)	1 or 2 softgels, 4 to 6 days per week	With fatty meals	Heart, bone health, and more. Prevents and removes calcification of the arteries
Jarrow Formulas—Zinc Balance (15 mg)	1 capsule 3 to 5 days a week	Between meals or with animal protein	Immune System, metabolism, weight loss, testosterone, asthma and more
LL's Magnetic Clay Nascent iodine (atomic iodine) (400 mcg per drop) (optional)	1 drop, 1 or 2 nonconsecutive days a week	Between meals with water	Metabolism, fatigue, depression, cancer, immune system, testosterone, heart disease, hair loss and more
Swanson—Buffered Chelated Magnesium Glycinate (133 mg)	100 to 400 mg per night, 30–60 minutes before bedtime	Empty stomach	Muscle cramps, heart health, bone health, blood pressure, weight loss, diabetes, migraines, ADHD and more
Solgar—Taurine (500 mg), Jarrow Formulas—Taurine (1,000 mg)	500–1000 mg before bedtime (with magnesium)	Empty stomach	Virtually every cellular function that keeps you alive
Potassium gluconate or citrate powder	400 to 800 mg a day (broken up between 2 to 4 separate doses)	With meals	Virtually every cellular function that keeps you healthy and alive
Nutrigold—Vitamin D3 (2000 mg)(5000 mg)	1 softgel, 2 (5000 IU) or 4 (2000 IU) days per week	With fatty meals	Heart, bone, muscle, immune system, more
Optimum Nutrition—Opti-Men/Opti-Women multivitamins	Opti-Men, 1 and 1/2 per day, or Opti-Women, 1 per day	With meals	Overall health. Try any of the top 25 brands listed at: MultivitaminGuide.Org
Citracal Petites (200 mg calcium citrate with D3)	1 or 2 tablets 3 to 5 days per week	With or without meals	Heart, bone, muscle, nerve health
GNC—Gentlesorb Iron (18 mg)	1 capsule any 1 to 3 days per week	Between meals, or with protein	Meat contains heme iron

Table 17. Carbohydrate, Protein, and Fiber Powders

Optimum Nutrition—Whey Protein (Gold Standard)	½ scoop with 2 scoops carb powder and ½ scoop of fiber in 1 percent milk at least 5 days per week (Preferably first thing in morning) Note: milk contains protein and carbs. Therefore full servings are not needed.	Between meals, or part of meal replacement	Consume 0.4 to 0.6 grams of protein for every pound of body weight. Include 1 to 2 grams of carb for every 1 gram of protein
Cytomax—Cyto Carb2 (mixes well with most beverages) or other carb powder	½ serving of carb powder with ½ serving protein and ½ serving of fiber in one percent milk at least 3 days per week (Preferably first thing in morning) Note: milk contains protein and carbs. Therefore full servings are not needed.	Between meals, or part of meal replacement	Carbohydrates are your body's and your brain's favorite and most efficient energy source
Garden of Life—Super Seed Beyond Fiber, (600 Grams)	According to the manufacturer's label, Super Seed can be mixed in smoothies, vegetable or fruit juice, cereal, yogurt or soup.	With meals or part of meal replacement	Try taking up to one serving a day, three to five days per week. Also, consume fiber-rich food. You must find ways to obtain adequate fiber daily

Nutrient Retention (in Cooked Food)

The United States Department of Agriculture (USDA) Table of Nutrient Retention Factors[i] is the major source of nutrient retention data for US and international food composition databases. The tables contain retention factors for 16 vitamins, 8 minerals, and alcohol for approximately 290 foods.

Most public and private-sector databases use USDA retention factors to calculate nutrient values when analytical data for cooked foods are unavailable. The resulting values indicate the nutrient content retained in a food after losses due to heating or other food preparation steps.

The following tables do not indicate the total amount (g, mg, IU, etc.) of a nutrient that is retained in the food item. The values represent the level of each nutrient that remains present in the food item after cooking. Basically, the values should be viewed in a similar fashion as percentages.

As indicated in the following tables, nutrients are very resilient to moderate heat. This is especially true of minerals and fat-soluble vitamins. When you boil food, however, much of the nutrient content transfers to the liquid (broth). If you do not drink the broth, you will lose that portion of the nutrients.

Only two of fourteen available nutrient retention tables were included here as an example of nutrient retention in cooked foods.

Additional information is available at www.notthecans.com/info/.

[i] Source: Nutrient Data Laboratory, Beltsville Human Nutrition Research Center (BHNRC), Agricultural Research Service (ARS), U.S. Department of Agriculture (USDA). Dec 2007.

Table 18. Nutrient Levels Retained in Food after Heating

Retention Description	Calcium, Ca	Iron, Fe	Magnesium, Mg	Phosphorus, P	Potassium, K	Sodium, Na	Zinc, Zn	Copper, Cu	Vitamin C, total ascorbic acid	Thiamin	Riboflavin	Niacin	Vitamin B-6	Folate, food	Folic acid	Folate, total	Choline, total	Vitamin B-12	Vitamin A, IU	Vitamin A, RE	Alcoh
CHEESE,BAKED	100	100	100	100	100	100	100	65	75	100	100	75	80	80	80	75	55	100	100	100	
CHEESE,BROILED	100	100	100	100	100	100	100	65	75	100	100	75	80	80	80	75	55	100	100	100	
CHEESE,COOKED W/LIQUID	100	100	100	100	100	100	100	65	75	100	100	75	80	80	80	75	55	100	100	100	
CHEESE,REHEATED	100	100	100	100	100	100	100	95	95	100	100	95	95	95	95	95	95	100	100	100	
EGGS,BAKED	100	100	100	100	100	100	100	80	80	95	90	95	75	75	75	80	80	100	100	100	
EGGS,FRIED,SCRAMBLED	100	100	100	100	100	100	100	80	85	95	95	95	75	75	75	85	85	100	100	100	
EGGS,HARD COOKED	100	100	100	100	100	100	100	80	85	95	95	95	75	75	75	80	85	100	100	100	
EGGS,POACHED	100	100	100	100	100	100	100	80	80	85	95	85	75	75	75	80	80	100	100	100	
EGGS,REHEATED	100	100	100	100	100	100	100	95	95	100	100	95	95	95	95	85	95	100	100	100	
MILK,HEATED APPROX 10MIN	100	100	100	100	100	100	100	85	90	100	100	90	85	85	85	90	80	100	100	100	
MILK,HEATED APPROX 30MIN	100	100	100	100	100	100	100	65	75	100	100	75	80	80	80	75	55	100	100	100	
MILK,HEATED APPROX 1 HOUR	100	100	100	100	100	100	100	45	60	100	100	55	70	70	70	60	30	100	100	100	
MILK,REHEATED	100	100	100	100	100	100	100	95	95	100	100	95	95	95	95	95	95	100	100	100	
CHICKEN,BROILED	95	90	75	80	80	100	95	80	70	90	80	80	60	60	60	70	65	75	75	75	
CHICKEN,FRIED,WO/COATING	95	90	75	80	80	100	95	80	70	90	80	80	60	60	60	70	65	75	75	75	
CHICKEN,FRIED,W/COATING	95	90	75	80	80	100	95	80	70	90	80	80	60	60	60	70	65	75	75	75	
CHICKEN,ROASTED	95	90	75	80	80	100	95	80	70	90	80	80	60	60	60	70	65	75	75	75	
CHICKEN,BROWN,SIMMER,WO/DRIPPINGS	80	90	65	60	70	100	90	80	55	95	60	50	60	60	60	70	50	75	75	75	
CHICKEN,BROWN,SIMMER,W/DRIPPINGS	100	100	100	100	100	100	100	85	75	100	95	95	70	70	70	70	65	80	80	80	
CHICKEN,SIMMERED,WO/DRIPPINGS	80	90	65	60	70	100	90	80	55	95	60	50	60	60	60	70	50	80	80	80	
CHICKEN,SIMMERED,W/DRIPPINGS	100	100	100	100	100	100	100	85	75	100	95	95	70	70	70	70	65	80	80	80	
CHICKEN,REHEATED	100	100	100	100	100	100	100	95	95	100	95	95	95	95	95	70	95	100	80	80	
TURKEY,ROASTED	100	95	80	75	75	100	70	80	65	85	90	70	60	60	60	70	65	75	100	100	

Table 18. Nutrient Levels Retained in Food after Heating (cont'd)

Retention Description	Calcium, Ca	Iron, Fe	Magnesium, Mg	Phosphorus, P	Potassium, K	Sodium, Na	Zinc, Zn	Copper, Cu	Vitamin C, total ascorbic acid	Thiamin	Riboflavin	Niacin	Vitamin B-6	Folate, food	Folic acid	Folate, total	Choline, total	Vitamin B-12	Vitamin A, IU	Vitamin A, RE	Alcoh
TURKEY,SIMMERED,WO/DRIPPINGS	85	95	65	70	55	70	100	95	80	55	95	60	50	60	60	60	70	50	75	75	100
TURKEY,SIMMERED,W/DRIPPINGS	100	100	100	100	100	100	100	100	85	75	100	95	70	70	70	70	70	70	80	80	100
TURKEY,REHEATED	100	100	100	100	100	100	100	95	95	95	100	100	95	95	95	95	95	95	100	100	100
OATMEAL,INST,COOKED	100	100	100	100	100	100	100	90	90	90	95	95	100	100	100	100	100	100	100	100	100
OATMEAL,REG/QUICK,COOKED	100	95	100	95	95	100	100	80	80	90	90	90	70	70	70	70	70	70	90	90	100
CEREAL,INST,COOKED	100	100	100	100	100	100	100	90	90	95	95	95	100	100	100	100	100	100	100	100	100
CEREAL,REG/QUICK,COOKED	100	95	100	95	95	100	100	80	80	90	90	90	70	70	70	70	70	70	90	90	100
FRUITS,FRESH(NOT CITRUS),BAKED	95	100	100	100	90	100	100	90	80	95	90	90	60	60	60	60	100	70	85	85	100
FRUITS,FRESH(NOT CITRUS),BROILED	95	100	100	100	90	100	100	80	80	95	90	90	60	60	60	60	100	85	85	85	100
FRUITS,FRESH(NOT CITRUS),SAUTEED	95	100	100	100	90	100	100	70	80	90	90	90	50	50	50	50	100	75	75	75	100
FRUITS,CANNED	95	100	100	100	90	100	100	50	80	90	90	90	50	50	50	50	100	75	75	75	100
FRUITS,FRESH(NOT CITRUS),STEWED	95	100	100	100	90	100	100	70	80	90	90	90	50	50	50	50	100	75	75	75	100
FRUITS,FROZEN	95	100	100	100	90	100	100	70	95	95	100	100	95	95	95	95	100	95	95	95	100
FRUITS,FRESH(NOT CITRUS),REHEATED	100	100	100	100	100	100	100	95	95	95	100	100	95	95	95	95	100	95	95	95	100
FRUITS,DRIED	100	100	100	100	100	100	100	20	70	90	90	90	50	50	50	50	100	50	50	50	100
FRUITS(DRIED),BAKED	95	100	100	100	90	100	100	80	80	95	90	90	60	60	60	60	100	85	85	85	100
FRUITS(DRIED),SAUTEED	95	100	100	100	90	100	100	70	80	90	90	90	50	50	50	50	100	75	75	75	100
FRUITS(DRIED),STEWED	95	100	100	100	90	100	100	70	80	90	90	90	50	50	50	50	100	75	75	75	100
FRUITS(DRIED),REHEATED	100	100	100	100	100	100	100	95	95	95	100	100	95	95	95	95	100	95	95	95	100
FRUITS,CITRUS,CKD	100	100	100	100	100	100	100	95	95	95	100	100	70	70	70	70	100	95	95	95	100
PORK,FRESH,BROILED	75	80	90	85	85	90	100	80	70	100	80	95	85	85	85	85	90	95	75	75	100
PORK,FRESH,FRIED,WO/COATING	75	80	95	85	85	90	100	80	70	100	80	95	85	85	85	85	90	75	75	75	100
PORK,FRESH,FRIED,W/COATING	75	80	95	85	85	90	100	80	70	100	80	95	85	85	85	85	90	90	75	75	100

Congratulations!

You have been empowered to recognize and reverse key nutrient deficiencies that significantly affect your health, fitness, and performance. Here are a few tips and takeaways:

- ✓ Do not drink caffeinated beverages with main meals or supplements. They significantly impair the absorption of key nutrients.
- ✓ Be aware that mineral absorption is significantly impaired by meals containing high amounts of phytate.
- ✓ Replace olive oil with coconut oil for stovetop cooking. Coconut oil retains its properties at high temperatures, but olive oil does not.
- ✓ Maintain a journal for one week documenting everything you eat, drink, and supplement. Use this to assess your nutrient intake.
- ✓ High-quality supplements absorb extremely well when compared to low-quality brands. Therefore, less is needed to restore and maintain sufficient levels in your system.
- ✓ Optimize your body's utilization of vitamin D3 by not taking a stand-alone supplement every day. Your body adapts to daily intake.
- ✓ Consider the amount and variety of nutrients naturally obtained from meals when deciding if supplementation is right for you.
- ✓ Buy three, 7-day pill containers in different colors for morning, noon, and evening use. Prefill them with supplements each week.
- ✓ Avoid multivitamins, caffeinated beverages, and vitamin C in the late evening, as they can impair your sleep.
- ✓ It takes several years to develop chronic nutrient deficiencies in industrialized countries. It may take up to one year to reverse them. When your diet does not supply adequate amounts of critical nutrients, your tissues release their stores to keep you alive and functioning. They need time to replenish their supply. Flooding your system with nutrients over extended periods introduces additional risks. Be patient and consistent by taking moderate doses over time.
- ✓ If you have been megadosing on a supplement, gradually reduce the dosage and, if needed, the frequency of consumption.
- ✓ Ignore bloggers who try to persuade individuals to consume massive doses of vitamins and minerals (even if the blogger is an MD). Years later we often discover adverse effects from doing so.
- ✓ Avoid the "latest and greatest" faux-diet fad.
- ✓ Recommend *It's Not the Cans* to your health care providers.

✓ Recommend *It's Not the Cans* to your family and friends.

In the following chapters we will discuss a few of the most common diseases that plague men and women today. All but one of these devastating illnesses (osteoporosis) rank among the top ten causes of death.

The information is well written, very informative and easily understood. However, I am not its author.

The vast majority of the following information was obtained directly from public-domain sources such as the CDC, the National Institutes of Health, and the National Institutes of Mental Health. I may have changed a word or two, but the full credit belongs to these institutions and every one of their dedicated employees and external contributors. The research they have conducted, and the reports they have compiled are filled with valuable health-related information, recommendations, facts, and statistics.

To these unsung heroes working tirelessly on our behalf and those who support them I say "Well done!"

My contributions to their effort are three-fold: 1) I reviewed and compared information from a multitude of sources and gathered key points into one place for your convenience. 2) I prioritized and organized the information into a logical flow, hopefully resulting in a less complicated read. 3) I researched and identified key nutrients that have been shown in a variety of studies to prevent, reverse, or lessen the severity of debilitating diseases.

Mortality in the United States

Donna L. Hoyert PhD, is a health scientist at the Centers for Disease Control and Prevention's NCHS, Division of Vital Statistics, Mortality Statistics Branch. Dr. Hoyert published the following information:[i]

> Since mortality statistics do not change markedly from year to year, one might not appreciate the progress in reducing mortality when looking at short-term change. This report uses data from the National Vital Statistics System (NVSS) over a 75-year period, including preliminary data for 2010, to examine long-term trends in mortality in the United States by age, sex, and race.
>
> While the total number of deaths increased by 1.1 million between 1935 and 2010, the risk of dying decreased. The crude death rate fell 27 percent from 1,094.5 to 798.7 deaths per 100,000 population between 1935 and 2010. The improvement in the risk of dying was actually larger than 27 percent because the U.S. population was getting older over this time period. When the effect of the aging of the population is removed by calculating an age-adjusted death rate, the risk of dying decreased by 60 percent from 1935 to 2010.
>
> Although there were year to year exceptions, the last 75 years witnessed sustained declines in the risk of dying in the United States.
>
> Between 1935 and 2010, age-adjusted death rates decreased by 56 percent for males and 62 percent for females.

Dr. Hoyert's report further establishes that the risk of dying decreased at a greater rate for younger age groups with a 94 percent reduction in death rates (on average) for individuals 1–4 years of age compared with a 38 percent decrease (on average) for individuals 85 years or older.

The report also states, "Heart disease, cancer, and stroke were among the five leading causes of death every year between 1935 and 2010." This remains true even today . . .

[i] Hoyert DL. "75 years of mortality in the United States, 1935–2010 NCHS data brief", last updated March 12, 2012, http://www.cdc.gov/nchs/data/databriefs/db88.htm

Nutrients That Prevent Heart Disease and Stroke

Fiber, Magnesium, Vitamin K2, Zinc, Taurine, Potassium, Omega-3, CoQ10

Heart disease is the leading cause of death among women and men. The most common type of heart disease within the United States is coronary artery disease (CAD), which can result in a heart attack. CAD occurs when cholesterol deposits (plaque) build up in arteries that supply blood to your heart. Calcium deposits then harden the plaque exacerbating the problem.

Heart Disease (Good News)

From a safety inspector's outlook, risk should be regarded in two aspects: likelihood and severity. Likelihood, in this instance, refers to how likely you are to develop heart disease. Severity is the level of adverse impact heart disease may have once it develops. Moderate physical activity helps to maintain a healthy heart. Balanced nutrition can reduce the likelihood of developing heart disease. It can also reduce the severity if it does develop. Of course, genetics and environmental factors also impacts heart health.

Heart Disease (More Good News)[i]

- ✓ Fiber lowers LDL cholesterol levels, enhances weight loss and it also lowers blood pressure in people with high blood pressure.
- ✓ Magnesium is critical to normal heart function. It regulates heart rhythm and lowers blood pressure.
- ✓ Vitamin K2 prevents and reduces hardening of the arteries.
- ✓ Zinc plays a defensive role in CAD and cardiomyopathy.
- ✓ Taurine improves heart function after congestive heart failure (CHF).
- ✓ Potassium is critical for heart function and normal heart rhythm.
- ✓ Omega-3 alpha-linolenic acid, eicosapentaenoic acid, and docosahexaenoic acid reduce risk of developing CAD. However, excessive fish oil intake may introduce other health risks[ii]
- ✓ CoQ10 may lower the risk of developing cardiovascular disease.

[i] Refer to corresponding chapters for additional details and references.
[ii] "Fish Oil Linked to Prostate Cancer Risk", September 3, 2013, http://www.nlm.nih.gov/medlineplus/podcast/transcript090313.html

Nutrients That Prevent Diabetes

Fiber, Magnesium, Potassium, Vitamin K2, Taurine, Potassium

According to the CDC,[i] 29.1 million people (9.3% of the US population) have diabetes, which is one of the leading causes of death among women and men. Roughly 21 million people have been diagnosed with diabetes, but there are an estimated 8.1 million people with the disease that have not been diagnosed. Diabetes is the leading cause of kidney failure, nontraumatic lower-limb amputations, and new cases of blindness among adults in the United States. It is also a major cause of heart disease and stroke.

At one time, type 2 diabetes was more common in people over forty-five. But now more young people have the disease due to weight.

Table 19. 2009–2012 National Health and Nutrition Examination Survey

	Number with diabetes (millions)	Percentage with diabetes (unadjusted)
Total		
20 years or older	28.9	12.3
By age		
20–44	4.3	4.1
45–64	13.4	16.2
65 years or older	11.2	25.9
By sex		
Men	15.5	13.6
Women	13.4	11.2

In 2009–2012, based on fasting glucose or A1C levels, 37% of U.S. adults aged 20 years or older had prediabetes (51% of those aged 65 years or older). In total, there are an estimated 86 million Americans aged 20 years or older with prediabetes.

The percentage of adults in the US aged 20 years or older with prediabetes was similar for non-Hispanic whites (35%), non-Hispanic blacks (39%), and Hispanics (38%).

Diabetes (Good News)

According to the National Diabetes Education Program (NDEP)[i], diabetes prevention is proven, possible, and powerful.

- Get at least thirty minutes of moderate-intensity physical activity five days a week.
- Eat a variety of foods that are low in fat. Reduce the number of calories you eat per day.

When you take steps to prevent diabetes, you will also lower your risk for possible complications from diabetes, such as heart disease, stroke, kidney disease, nerve damage, and other health problems.

Diabetes (More Good News)[ii]

- ✓ Dietary fiber lowers the risk of diabetes and enhances weight loss.
- ✓ Magnesium significantly improves insulin sensitivity and normal cell function for diabetics. It also lowers risk of type 2 diabetes.
- ✓ Vitamin K2 supplementation improves insulin sensitivity.
- ✓ Zinc is beneficial to glycemic control metabolism and immune function.
- ✓ Taurine reduces blood glucose and restores insulin sensitivity.
- ✓ Potassium is a double-edged sword for diabetes. Maintaining proper levels lowers the risk for developing diabetes. However, individuals with diabetes may develop unsafe, high-levels of potassium due to impaired kidney function and therefore should consult with their physician. As stated earlier, there are an estimated 8.1 million people with diabetes that have not been diagnosed.

[i] Established in 1997, the National Diabetes Education Program is a federally-funded program sponsored by the U.S. Department of Health and Human Services' National Institutes of Health and the CDC: http://ndep.nih.gov

[ii] Please refer to corresponding nutrient chapters for additional details and references.

Nutrients That Prevent Osteoporosis

Magnesium, Vitamin D, Calcium, Vitamin K2, Zinc, Taurine

According to the National Institutes of Health,[1] osteoporosis (porous bone) is a disease characterized by low bone mass and structural deterioration of bone tissue, leading to bone fragility and an increased risk of fractures of the hip, spine, and wrist. Both men and women are affected by osteoporosis, a disease that can be prevented and treated. In the United States, more than 40 million people already have osteoporosis or are at high risk due to low bone mass.

A National Health and Nutrition Examination Survey[2] conducted from 2005–2008 determined that 9 percent of adults aged fifty years and over had osteoporosis, as defined by the World Health Organization.

The prevalence of osteoporosis or low bone mass differs by age, sex, and ethnicity. Women are at greater risk of developing this disease. The likelihood increases with age.

Figure 3. Adults 50+: Osteoporosis or Low Bone Mass by Age

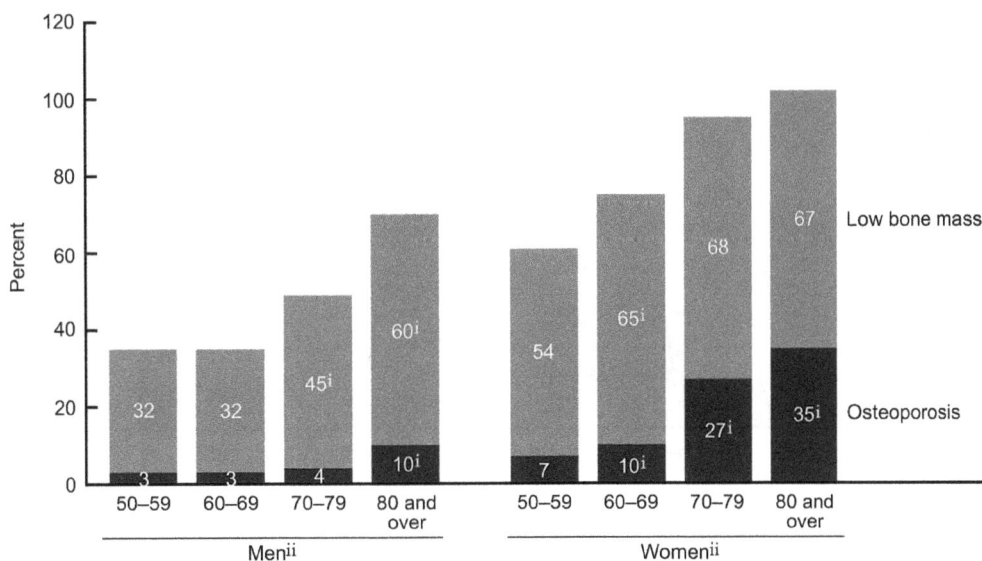

CDC/NCHS, National Health and Nutrition Examination Survey, 2005–2008[i],[ii]

[i] $p < 0.05$ compared with preceding age group within sex and skeletal status category.
[ii] $p < 0.05$ for trend by age group within sex for both osteoporosis and low bone mass.

Figure 4. Women 50+: Osteoporosis or Low Bone Mass by Ethnicity

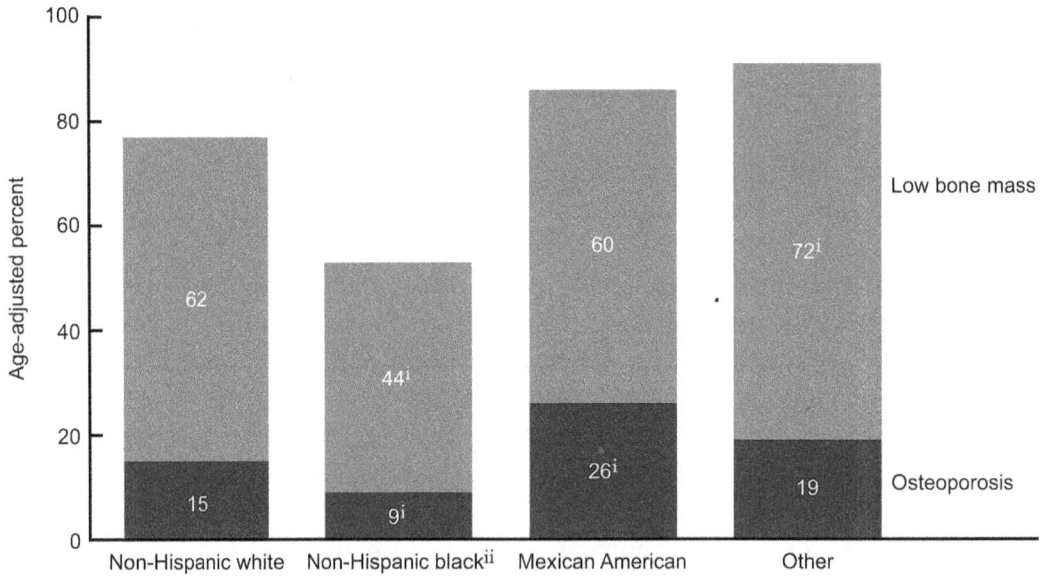

CDC/NCHS, National Health and Nutrition Examination Survey, 2005–2008

Figure 5. Men 50+: Osteoporosis or Low Bone Mass by Ethnicity

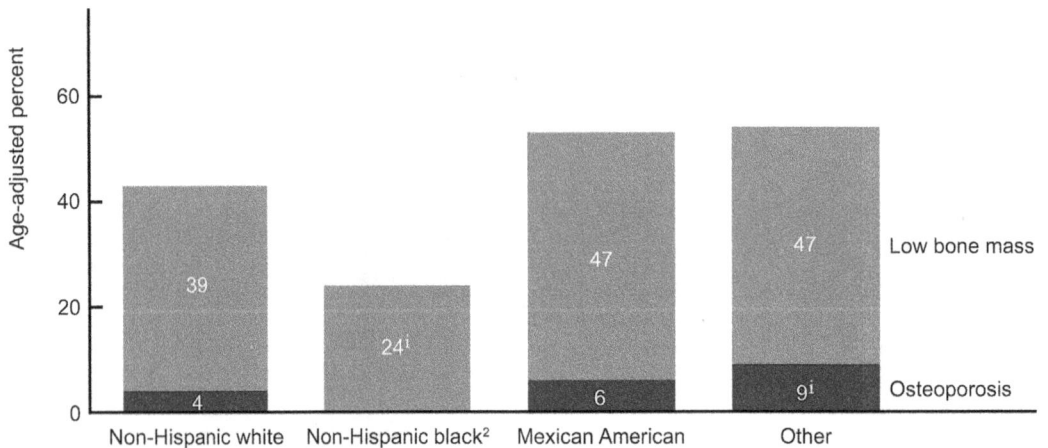

CDC/NCHS, National Health and Nutrition Examination Survey, 2005–2008

Osteoporosis (Good News)

Preventing osteoporosis is very doable. Proper nutrition and exercise are key factors in maintaining bone health. Attaining your body's peak bone mass and minimizing bone loss as you grow older is a lifelong commitment. There are a multitude of factors to consider regarding long-term bone health. Comprehensively addressing all these factors drastically reduces your likelihood of developing osteoporosis.

Bone is living tissue that responds to exercise by becoming stronger. Physical activity early in life contributes to higher peak bone mass. Excessive exercise, however, can be bad for bone health. The best exercise for building and maintaining bone mass is weight-bearing exercise: exercise that you do on your feet and that forces you to work against gravity, such as jogging, aerobics, hiking, walking, stair climbing, gardening, weight training, resistance training, tennis, and dancing.

Experts recommend thirty minutes or more of moderate physical activity on most (preferably all) days of the week, including a mix of weight-bearing exercises, strength training (two or three times a week), and balance training.

Taking steps to prevent osteoporosis, will also lower your risk of developing diabetes, heart disease, and other chronic health problems.

Osteoporosis (More Good News)[i]

- ✓ Magnesium activates vitamin D to absorb calcium. It is also one of the building blocks for bone structure and density.
- ✓ Vitamin D gives you the ability to absorb large amounts of calcium.
- ✓ Calcium is a core building block for bones, teeth, and other tissues.
- ✓ Vitamin K2 activates proteins that bind calcium to your bones.
- ✓ Potassium intake is directly associated with bone mineral density.
- ✓ Zinc has a restorative effect on bone loss and increases bone mass.
- ✓ Taurine enhances bone tissue formation and retards bone loss.

---

[1] "Osteoporosis", accessed July 2014, http://www.niams.nih.gov/Health_Info/Bone/Osteoporosis/default.asp

[2] Looker AC, Borrud LC, Dawson-Hughes B, et al. (2012 Apr). Osteoporosis or Low Bone Mass at the Femur Neck or Lumbar Spine in Older Adults: United States, 2005–2008. *NCHS Data Brief.* No. 93

[i] Refer to corresponding chapters for additional details and references.

Nutrients That Prevent Depression

Zinc, Magnesium, Taurine, Vitamin D, Multivitamins, Iodine, CoQ10

Depression is a multifaceted illness that too often goes ignored. Anyone who has suffered from depression fully understands how deep and paralyzing its effects can be. Depression can occur for a variety of reasons, including hormonal imbalances, financial hardships, and psychological or physical abuse.

The following information was obtained directly from the National Institute of Mental Health (NIMH).[i]

How Do Women Experience Depression?

Depression is more common among women than among men. Biological, life cycle, hormonal, and psychosocial factors that women experience may be linked to women's higher depression rate. Researchers have shown that hormones directly affect the brain chemistry that controls emotions and mood. For example, women are especially vulnerable to developing depression after giving birth, when hormonal and physical changes and the new responsibility of caring for a newborn can be overwhelming.

Some women may also have a severe form of premenstrual syndrome (PMS) called premenstrual dysphoric disorder (PMDD). PMDD is associated with the hormonal changes that typically occur around ovulation and before menstruation begins.

During the transition into menopause, some women experience an increased risk for depression. In addition, osteoporosis may be associated with depression. Scientists are exploring all of these potential connections and how the cyclical rise and fall of estrogen and other hormones may affect a woman's brain chemistry.

Finally, many women face the additional stresses of work and home responsibilities, caring for children and aging parents, abuse, poverty, and relationship strains. It is still unclear, though, why some women faced with enormous challenges develop depression while others with similar challenges do not.[ii]

---

[i] The National Institute of Mental Health (NIMH) is part of the National Institutes of Health (NIH), a component of the U.S. Department of Health and Human Services.

[ii] Author's note: Nutrient disparities may be one of several factors in why people respond differently under extremely challenging circumstances.

How Do Men Experience Depression?

Men often experience depression differently from women. Women with depression are more likely to have feelings of sadness, worthlessness, and excessive guilt. Men are more likely to be very tired, irritable, and introverted; lose interest in once-pleasurable activities; and have difficulty sleeping.

Men may be more likely than women to turn to alcohol or drugs when they are depressed. They also may become frustrated, discouraged, short-tempered, angry, and sometimes abusive. Some men throw themselves into their work to avoid talking about their depression with family or friends, or behave recklessly. And although more women attempt suicide, many more men die by suicide in the United States.

How Do Older Adults Experience Depression?

Depression is not a normal part of aging. Most seniors feel satisfied with their lives, despite having more illnesses or physical problems. However, when older adults do have depression, it may be overlooked because seniors may show different, less obvious symptoms. Some seniors may be less likely to display or admit to feelings of sadness or grief.

Sometimes it can be difficult to distinguish grief from major depression. Grief after loss of a loved one is a normal reaction to the loss and generally does not require professional mental health treatment. However, grief that is complicated and lasts for a very long time following a loss may require treatment. Researchers continue to study the relationship between complicated grief and major depression.

Older adults also may have more medical conditions such as heart disease, stroke, or cancer, which may cause depressive symptoms. Or they may be taking medications with side effects that contribute to depression. Some older adults may experience what doctors call vascular depression, also called arteriosclerotic depression or subcortical ischemic depression. Vascular depression may result when blood vessels become less flexible and harden over time, becoming constricted. Such hardening of vessels prevents normal blood flow to the body's organs, including the brain. Those with vascular depression may have, or be at risk for, co-existing heart disease or stroke.

Although many people assume that the highest rates of suicide are among young people, white males age 85 and older actually have the highest suicide rate in the United States. Many have a depressive illness that their doctors are not aware of, even though many of these suicide victims visit their doctors within one month of their deaths.

The majority of older adults with depression improve when they receive treatment with an antidepressant, psychotherapy, or a combination of both. Research has shown that medication alone and combination treatment are both effective in reducing depression in older adults. Psychotherapy alone can also be effective in helping older adults stay free of depression, especially among those with minor depression. Psychotherapy is particularly useful for those who are unable or unwilling to take antidepressant medication.

How Can I Help a Loved One Who Is Depressed?

If you know someone who is depressed, it affects you too. The most important thing you can do is help the individual to get a diagnosis and treatment. You may need to make an appointment and go with him or her to see the doctor. Encourage your loved one to stay in treatment, or to seek different treatment if no improvement occurs after six to eight weeks.

To Help Your Friend or Relative

- ✓ Offer emotional support, understanding, patience, and encouragement.
- ✓ Talk to him or her, and listen carefully.
- ✓ Never dismiss feelings, but point out realities and offer hope.
- ✓ Never ignore comments about suicide, and report them to your loved one's therapist or doctor.
- ✓ Invite your loved one out for walks, outings and other activities. Keep trying if he or she declines, but don't push him or her to take on too much too soon.
- ✓ Provide assistance in getting to doctor's appointments.
- ✓ Remind your loved one that with time and treatment, the depression will lift.

How Can I Help Myself if I am Depressed?

If you have depression, you may feel exhausted, helpless, and hopeless. It may be extremely difficult to take any action to help yourself. But as you begin to recognize your depression and begin treatment, you will start to feel better.

To Help Yourself

- ✓ Do not wait too long to get evaluated or treated. There is research showing the longer one waits, the greater the impairment can be down the road. Try to see a professional as soon as possible.

- ✓ Try to be active and exercise. Go to a movie, a ballgame, or another event or activity that you once enjoyed.
- ✓ Set realistic goals for yourself.
- ✓ Break up large tasks into small ones, set some priorities, and do what you can as you can.
- ✓ Try to spend time with other people and confide in a trusted friend or relative. Try not to isolate yourself, and let others help you.
- ✓ Expect your mood to improve gradually, not immediately. Do not expect to suddenly "snap out of" your depression. Often during treatment for depression, sleep and appetite will begin to improve before your depressed mood lifts.
- ✓ Postpone important decisions, such as getting married or divorced or changing jobs, until you feel better. Discuss decisions with others who know you well and have a more objective view of your situation.
- ✓ Remember that positive thinking will replace negative thoughts as your depression responds to treatment.
- ✓ Continue to educate yourself about depression

For more details, please visit the National Institute of Mental Health (NIMH) at: http://www.nimh.nih.gov/health/topics/depression/

Depression (Good News)[i]

- ✓ Zinc mitigates and helps reverse some forms of depression.
- ✓ Magnesium relieves depression.
- ✓ L-taurine deficiency increases the risk for depression.
- ✓ Vitamin D deficiency significantly can cause or worsen depression.
- ✓ Multivitamins have a restorative effect on appetite and energy. They also a good source of B-complex vitamins such as B9 (Folic Acid). B vitamin deficiency can trigger or worsen depression.
- ✓ Iodine deficiency has been linked to depression.
- ✓ CoQ10 appears to benefit individuals who suffer from depression.

Nutrient balance can prevent, and even help reverse some forms of depression. It can also alleviate related symptoms such as fatigue.

---

[i] Refer to corresponding chapters for additional details and references.

Nutrients That Prevent Obesity

Fiber, Magnesium, Potassium, Vitamin K2, Taurine, Potassium

According to the CDC[i], in 1990, among states participating in the Behavioral Risk Factor Surveillance System, 10 states had a prevalence of obesity less than 10% and no state had prevalence equal to or greater than 15%.

By 2000, no state had a prevalence of obesity less than 10%, 23 states had prevalence between 20–24%, and no state had prevalence equal to or greater than 25%.

In 2010, no state had a prevalence of obesity less than 20%. Thirty-six states had a prevalence equal to or greater than 25%; 12 of these states (Alabama, Arkansas, Kentucky, Louisiana, Michigan, Mississippi, Missouri, Oklahoma, South Carolina, Tennessee, Texas, and West Virginia) had a prevalence equal to or greater than 30%.

Figure 6. 2010 Obesity Rates among U.S. Adults by State ii

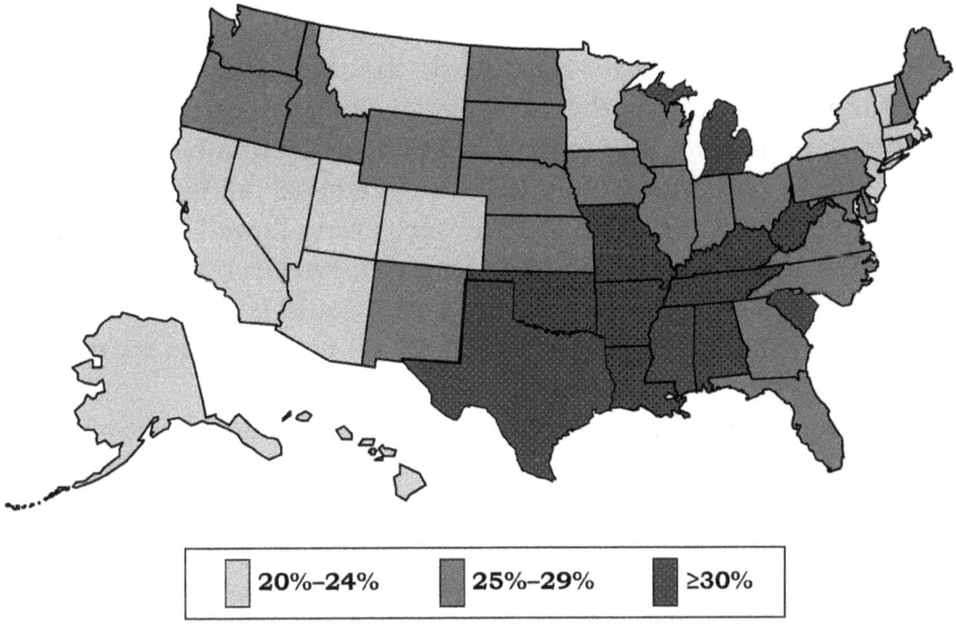

20%–24%   25%–29%   ≥30%

---

[i] CDC Obesity Trends Among U.S. Adults Between 1985 and 2010 http://www.cdc.gov/obesity/downloads/obesity_trends_2010.ppt

[ii] CDC Behavioral Risk Factor Surveillance System (BRSS).

As stated in a 1998 National Institutes of Health publication [1] (No. 98-4083), an estimated 97 million adults in the United States [at that time] are overweight or obese, substantially raising their risk of morbidity from hypertension, dyslipidemia, type 2 diabetes, coronary heart disease, stroke, gallbladder disease, osteoarthritis, sleep apnea and respiratory problems, and endometrial, breast, prostate, and colon cancers. Higher body weights are also associated with increases in all-cause mortality. Overweight and obesity pose a major public health challenge in the United States. Overweight is defined as a body mass index (BMI) of 25 to 29.9 kg/m2 and obesity as a BMI of [3] 30 kg/m2

As indicated by the National Center for Health Statistics [2], 27.4% of men with a college degree are obese compared with 32.1% of men with less than a high school education. Statistically, this difference is not significant. However, among women, 23.4% of women with a college degree are obese, compared to 42.1% of women with less than a high school education that are obese. As a data analyst, I can't help but ponder the psychological, cultural, and physiological implications of these findings.

It is fairly obvious that weight management has become more challenging. It isn't due to any single issue, rather a myriad of issues. Prior to gaming consoles and cable TV, one could argue that individuals were more active. Prior to self-propelled lawnmowers, electric hedge trimmers, leaf blowers and the like, yard-work was hard-work that required a lot of energy. I even recall watching my mother scrub clothes and linen on a scrub-board and hanging them on a line to dry. In the absence of a heavy rain storm, going outside to play was a daily treat. In grade school we were given two recess periods a day to run about. We were even allowed to walk home for lunch. Before the computer and the internet, research required a trip to the library (versus hitting the "on" button). I could go on but I believe the point has been made. People today simply do not burn as many calories per month like we use to (mainly because we had to).

In addition, sugary foods were a treat versus a major part of our daily cuisine. Many neighborhoods had local grocery stores that sold fresh produce that was not genetically modified, chemically enhanced, or overly processed. Most meals were cooked at home and not premade or obtained from drive-through windows. Meats were obtained from a butcher versus the high sodium, frozen-food section.

I am not advocating against advances in technology. I am sharing examples of changes that have occurred in my lifetime that directly affect weight management. Nutrient balance can play an integral role in combatting obesity.

Yet it is often overlooked. Rarely, if ever, is an individual struggling with weight management asked, "Are you getting enough zinc? How about magnesium?" These and other nutrients play a critical role in metabolic processes. Nutrient balance alone is not a cure for obesity. It is, however, a very effective strategy that can greatly enhance your efforts to maintain a healthy weight.

Obesity (Good News)

Obesity can be prevented and even reversed. Proper nutrition, physical activity, stress management, and weight monitoring are all proven to prevent and reverse excessive weight gain.

When you take steps to prevent gaining excessive weight, you will also lower your risk for developing diabetes, heart disease, stroke, cancer, and other health problems.

Obesity (More Good News) [i]

Regardless of your lifestyle and your diet, adequate (not excessive) levels of key nutrients are extremely beneficial to weight loss and weight management. Nutrient balance is not a single solution. It is a key player in your comprehensive approach toward better weight management. Always consider, more is not better. Balance is what your body craves.

- ✓ Dietary fiber (not a nutrient) significantly enhances weight loss.
- ✓ Magnesium lowers the level of fasting glucose and insulin. It is a key component to multiple weight-management metabolic functions.
- ✓ Zinc is very beneficial to metabolism. Obese individuals typically present significantly lower than normal zinc levels.
- ✓ Vitamin D supports weight-loss.
- ✓ Taurine burns fat, slows weight gain and promotes weight loss.
- ✓ Potassium helps build muscle and burn carbohydrates for energy.
- ✓ Iodine maintains thyroid health, which regulates metabolism.

[1]   Clinical Guidelines on the Identification, Evaluation, and Treatment of Overweight and Obesity in Adults: The Evidence Report, a http://www.nhlbi.nih.gov/health-pro/guidelines/archive/obesity-guidelines/full-report.htm

[2]   Ogden CL, Lamb MM, Carroll MD, Flegal KM. (2010 Dec) Obesity and socioeconomic status in adults: United States 2005–2008. *NCHS Data Brief.* :50. http://www.cdc.gov/nchs/data/databriefs/db50.pdf

[i]   Refer to corresponding chapters for additional details and references.

Nutrients That May Prevent Breast Cancer

Iodine, Magnesium, Vitamin D

According to the CDC[i], breast cancer is the most common cancer among American women. The different forms of breast cancer are categorized according to which cells in the breast develop into cancer. Breast cancer can begin in different parts of the breast, such as the ducts or the lobes. Breast cancer occurs in both men and women, though male breast cancer is rare. Radiation exposure, high levels of estrogen, and a family history of breast cancer can increase a man's risk of breast cancer.

Estimated new cases and deaths from breast cancer in the United States in 2014: [ii]

- New cases: 232,670 (female); 2,360 (male)
- Deaths: 40,000 (female); 430 (male)

Symptoms

Different people have different warning signs for breast cancer. Some people do not have any signs or symptoms at all. Some symptoms of breast cancer are:

- ❑ New lump in the breast or underarm (armpit)
- ❑ Thickening or swelling of part of the breast
- ❑ Irritation or dimpling of breast skin
- ❑ Redness or flaky skin in the nipple area or the breast
- ❑ Pulling in of the nipple or pain in the nipple area
- ❑ Nipple discharge other than breast milk, including blood
- ❑ Any change in the size or the shape of the breast
- ❑ Pain in any area of the breast

If you have any symptoms that worry you, be sure to see your doctor right away.

[i] Source: *Division of Cancer Prevention and Control, National Center for Chronic Disease Prevention and Health Promotion:* www.cdc.gov/CANCER/breast/basic_info

[ii] Source: National Cancer Institute (NCI) Estimated new cases and deaths from prostate cancer in the United States in 2014: http://www.cancer.gov/cancertopics/types/breast

Breast Cancer (Good News)

Having regular mammograms can lower the risk of mortality from breast cancer. From ages fifty to seventy-four, be sure to have a screening mammogram every two years. If you are between forty and forty-nine years old, talk to your doctor about a screening mammogram.

You can lower your risk of breast cancer in the following ways:

- Get screened for breast cancer regularly.
- Keep a healthy weight.
- Exercise regularly.
- Limit alcoholic drinks to no more than one per day.
- If you are taking, or have been told to take, hormone replacement therapy or oral contraceptives (birth control pills), ask your doctor about the risks.
- Breastfeed your babies if possible.

Please visit the National Cancer Institute (NCI) for more information. http://www.cancer.gov/cancertopics/types/breast

Breast Cancer (More Good News) [i]

- ✓ Iodine shrinks cancer cells, impedes cancer cellular activity, and causes apoptosis (automatic cell death) of cancer cells.
- ✓ Magnesium has been shown to lower the risk of developing cancer.
- ✓ Vitamin D supplements plus calcium may lower the risk of developing cancer of any type.

---

[i]   Refer to corresponding chapters for additional details and references.

Nutrients That May Prevent Prostate Cancer

Iodine, Magnesium, Vitamin D

According to the CDC,[i] except for skin cancer, prostate cancer is the most common cancer in American men. Many men with prostate cancer, especially with tumors that have not spread beyond the prostate, die of other causes without ever having any symptoms from the cancer itself.

As men age, the prostate tends to increase in size. This can cause the urethra to narrow and decrease urine flow. This is called benign prostatic hyperplasia, and it is not the same as prostate cancer.

Estimated new cases and deaths from prostate cancer in the United States in 2014: [ii]

- New cases: 233,000
- Deaths: 29,480

A man with a father, brother, or son who has had prostate cancer is two to three times more likely to develop the disease himself.

Symptoms

Different people have different symptoms for prostate cancer. Some men have no symptoms. Some symptoms of prostate cancer are:

- ❑ Difficulty starting urination
- ❑ Weak or interrupted urine flow
- ❑ Frequent urination, especially at night
- ❑ Difficulty emptying the bladder
- ❑ Pain or burning during urination
- ❑ Blood in the urine or semen
- ❑ Continuous pain in the back, hips, or pelvis
- ❑ Painful ejaculation

[i] Source: Division of Cancer Prevention and Control, National Center for Chronic Disease Prevention and Health Promotion: http://www.cdc.gov/CANCER/prostate/basic_info/
[ii] Source: National Cancer Institute (NCI) Estimated new cases and deaths from prostate cancer in the United States in 2014: http://www.cancer.gov/cancertopics/types/prostate

If you have any symptoms that worry you, see your doctor right away. Keep in mind that these symptoms may be caused by conditions other than prostate cancer.

Prostate Cancer (Good News)

In the United States from 2001 to 2010, prostate cancer decreased by:

- Caucasian men—4.0% per year.
- African American men—2.6% per year.
- Hispanic men—3.1% per year.
- Asian/Pacific Islander men—3.9% per year.

Prostate Cancer (More Good News) [i]

- ✓ Iodine shrinks cancer cells, impedes cancer cellular activity, and causes apoptosis (automatic cell death) of cancer cells.
- ✓ Magnesium lowered the risk of developing cancer in studies.
- ✓ Vitamin D supplementation may lower the risk of developing prostate cancer, especially among African Americans.[1]
- ✗ Vitamin E research [2] published October 12, 2011, in the Journal of American Medical Association concluded that the risk of prostate cancer among healthy men significantly increased at 400 IU of vitamin E supplementation.
- ✗ The National Library of Medicine [3] warns that men with higher levels of fish oil (or omega-3 fatty acids) in their blood have a 44 percent higher risk for developing prostate cancer. The message was prompted by a study [4] published by the National Cancer Institute.

Please be aware that there are ongoing discussions regarding these findings. Continue to update yourself on this issue as more data becomes available. If you take fish oil supplements, you are encouraged to do so in moderation (possibly 1 g or less). Also, consider not supplementing daily.

[i] Refer to corresponding chapters for additional details and references.

1 "Low Vitamin D Might Be Linked to Prostate Cancer", May 1, 2014, http://www. webmd.com/prostate-cancer/news/20140501/low-vitamin-d-linked-to-aggressive-advanced-prostate-cancers-study

2 Klein EA, Thompson IM Jr, Tangen CM, et al. (2011 Oct 12). Vitamin E and the risk of prostate cancer: the Selenium and Vitamin E Cancer Prevention Trial (SELECT). *JAMA*. 306(14):1549-56. doi: 10.1001/jama.2011.1437.

3 "Fish Oil Linked to Prostate Cancer Risk", September 3, 2013, http://www.nlm.nih. gov/medlineplus/podcast/transcript090313.html

4 Brasky TM, Darke AK, Song X, et al. (2011 Oct 12). Plasma Phospholipid Fatty Acids and Prostate Cancer Risk in the SELECT Trial. *J Natl Cancer Inst*. 105(15):1132-1141. doi: 10.1093/jnci/djt174

Women Leading Causes of Death

The information contained in the following tables was obtained from HHS, CDC, and NCHS. Portions of the tables have been removed.

Table 20. Leading Causes of Death: Females in United States, 2010

Caucasian	%*	African American	%*
1) Heart disease	23.5	1) Heart disease	24.1
2) Cancer	22	2) Cancer	22.6
3) Chronic lower resp. diseases	6.4	3) Stroke	6.4
4) Stroke	6.2	4) Diabetes	4.6
5) Alzheimer's disease	5	5) Kidney disease	3.4
6) Unintentional injuries	3.7	6) Chronic lower resp. diseases	3
7) Diabetes	2.4	7) Unintentional injuries	2.8
8) Influenza and pneumonia	2.2	8) Alzheimer's disease	2.6
9) Kidney disease	1.9	9) Septicemia	2.3
10) Septicemia	1.4	10) Hypertension	2.1
Asian or Pacific Islander	%*	**Hispanic**	%*
1) Cancer	28.3	1) Cancer	22.6
2) Heart disease	21.3	2) Heart disease	20.9
3) Stroke	8.5	3) Stroke	6
4) Diabetes	3.7	4) Diabetes	4.9
5) Unintentional injuries	3.3	5) Unintentional injuries	4.4
6) Alzheimer's disease	3	6) Alzheimer's disease	3.5
7) Influenza and pneumonia	2.9	7 Chronic lower resp. diseases	3.1
8) Chronic lower resp. diseases	2.3	8) Kidney disease	2.4
9) Kidney disease	2.3	9) Influenza and pneumonia	2.3
10) Hypertension	1.9	10) Chronic liver disease	2

* Percent (%) represents total percentages of deaths.

- FOR THE FOLLOWING TABLES -

Percentages represent total deaths in the age group due to the cause indicated. Numbers in parentheses indicate tied rankings. The white, black, American Indian/Alaska Native, and Asian/Pacific Islander race groups include persons of Hispanic and non-Hispanic origin who may be of any race. Some terms have been shortened from those used in the National Vital Statistics Report.

Refer to pages 134—135 for a listing of the shortened terms in the table and their full, unabridged equivalents used in the report.

Table 21. Women—Caucasian: Leading Causes of Death by Age Group—USA, 2010*

	Ages 15-19	20-24	25-34	35-44	45-54	55-64	65+
1	Accidental injuries 49.2%	Accidental injuries 45.3%	Accidental injuries 33.1%	Cancer 25.5%	Cancer 36.1%	Cancer 41.3%	Heart disease 25.8%
2	Suicide 12.1%	Suicide 11.2%	Cancer 14.4%	Accidental injuries 20.2%	Heart disease 13.8%	Heart disease 15.9%	Cancer 19.2%
3	Cancer 7.7%	Cancer 7.8%	Suicide 9.9%	Heart disease 10.7%	Accidental injuries 10.3%	Chronic lower resp. disease 6.3%	Stroke 6.9%
4	Homicide 5.2%	Homicide 5.8%	Heart disease 6.6%	Suicide 6.9%	Chronic liver disease 4.3%	Accidental injuries 3.9%	Chronic lower resp. diseases 6.8%
5	Heart disease 2.7%	Heart disease 3.0%	Homicide 4.0%	Chronic liver disease 3.3%	Chronic lower resp. diseases 3.7%	Diabetes 3.4%	Alzheimer's disease 6.1%
6	Birth defects 2.5%	Pregnancy complications 2.2%	Pregnancy complications 2.3%	Stroke 2.8%	Suicide 3.5%	Stroke 3.3%	Influenza and pneumonia 2.4%
7	Pregnancy complications 1.3%	Birth defects 1.7%	Stroke 1.8%	Diabetes 2.5%	Stroke 3.1%	Chronic liver disease 2.5%	Diabetes 2.4%

Table 22. Women—African American: Leading Causes of Death by Age Group—USA, 2010*

	Ages 15-19	20-24	25-34	35-44	45-54	55-64	65+
1	Accidental injuries 25.4%	Accidental injuries 24.7%	Accidental injuries 15.1%	Cancer 22.3%	Cancer 30.4%	Cancer 34.1%	Heart disease 27.2%
2	Homicide 22.3%	Homicide 14.5%	Heart disease 11.9%	Heart disease 17.8%	Heart disease 20.1%	Heart disease 22.5%	Cancer 20.2%
3	Cancer 8.8%	Heart disease 9.3%	Cancer 11.7%	Accidental injuries 8.4%	Stroke 5.5%	Diabetes 5.3%	Stroke 7.4%
4	Heart disease 6.0%	Cancer 6.9%	Homicide 9.4%	HIV disease 7.2%	Accidental injuries 5.1%	Stroke 5.3%	Diabetes 4.9%
5	Suicide 3.7%	Suicide 5.2%	HIV disease 6.9%	Stroke 4.6%	Diabetes 4.1%	Kidney disease 3.2%	Alzheimer disease 4.1%
6	Birth defects 2.7%	Pregnancy complications 4.1%	Pregnancy complications 4.1%	Diabetes 3.6%	HIV disease 3.7%	Chronic lower resp. diseases 3.1%	Kidney disease 3.9%
7	Stroke *** Chronic lower resp. diseases	HIV disease 3.4%	Diabetes 3.4%	Homicide 3.0%	Kidney disease 2.7%	Septicemia 2.5%	Chronic lower resp. diseases 3.3%

Table 23. Women—Asian or Pacific Islander: Leading Causes of Death by Age Group—USA, 2010*

	Ages 15-19	20-24	25-34	35-44	45-54	55-64	65+
1	Accidental injuries 33.0%	Accidental injuries 25.6%	Cancer 26.4%	Cancer 44.4%	Cancer 54.3%	Cancer 51.1%	Heart disease 25.2%
2	Suicide 18.7%	Suicide 22.2%	Accidental injuries 16.3%	Suicide 8.7%	Heart disease 8.3%	Heart disease 13.6%	Cancer 22.9%
3	Cancer 13.2%	Cancer 13.7%	Suicide 14.8%	Heart disease (3) 6.5% ***	Stroke 6.2%	Stroke 7.4%	Stroke 9.3%
4	Heart disease (4) 4.4% ***	Homicide 6.8%	Pregnancy complications 6.4%	Stroke (3) 6.5% ***	Accidental injuries 5.4%	Accidental injuries 3.5%	Diabetes 4.1%
5	Homicide (4) 4.4% ***	Heart disease 6.0%	Heart disease 6.2%	Accidental injuries (3) 6.5%	Suicide 3.7%	Diabetes 3.2%	Alzheimer's disease 4.0%
6	Anemias (6) 2.2% ***	Stroke 3.4%	Homicide 3.9%	Homicide 3.0%	Diabetes 2.5%	Kidney disease 2.0%	Influenza & pneumonia 3.5%
7	Birth defects (6) 2.2%	Birth defects 2.6%	Stroke 3.2%	Diabetes 2.7%	Chronic liver disease 1.6%	Suicide 1.6%	Chronic lower respiratory diseases 2.9%

Table 24. Women—Hispanic: Leading Causes of Death by Age Group—USA, 2010*

	Ages 15-19	20-24	25-34	35-44	45-54	55-64	65+
1	Accidental injuries 42.1%	Accidental injuries 34.1%	Accidental injuries 24.4%	Cancer 31.2%	Cancer 38.2%	Cancer 36.9%	Heart disease 26.0%
2	Suicide 14.1%	Cancer 11.8%	Cancer 21.5%	Accidental injuries 13.8%	Heart disease 12.7%	Heart disease 16.1%	Cancer 19.4%
3	Homicide 10.1%	Suicide 10.3%	Homicide 6.7%	Heart disease 8.3%	Accidental injuries 7.3%	Diabetes 6.3%	Stroke 7.1%
4	Cancer 9.2%	Homicide 9.6%	Suicide 5.4%	Stroke 4.2%	Chronic liver disease 5.5%	Stroke 4.9%	Diabetes 5.4%
5	Birth defects 2.7%	Pregnancy complication 4.2%	Heart disease 4.9%	Suicide 3.7%	Stroke 4.7%	Chronic liver disease 3.8%	Alzheimer's disease 5.1%
6	Heart disease 2.0%	Heart disease 3.5%	Pregnancy complication 4.5%	Diabetes 3.6%	Diabetes 4.1%	Accidental injuries 3.7%	Chronic lower resp. diseases 3.9%
7	Septicemia 0.9% *** Kidney disease 0.9%	Birth defects 2.0%	Stroke 2.0%	Chronic liver disease 3.4%	Chronic lower resp. diseases 1.7% *** Kidney disease 1.7%	Kidney disease 2.7%	Kidney disease 2.8%

Some terms in the leading causes of death tables have been shortened from those used in the National Vital Statistics Report. Below is a listing of the shortened terms used in the table and their full, unabridged equivalents used in the report.

Short Terms	Full Terms
Aortic aneurism	Aortic aneurism and dissection
Appendix disease	Diseases of appendix
Benign neoplasms	In situ neoplasms and neoplasms of uncertain or unknown behavior
Birth defects	Congenital malformations, deformations, and chromosomal abnormalities
Bronchitis	Acute bronchitis and bronchiolitis
Cancer	Malignant neoplasms
C. difficile infection	Entercolitis due to clostridium
Chronic liver disease	Chronic liver disease and cirrhosis
Chronic lower-respiratory diseases	Includes bronchitis, emphysema, asthma, bronchiectasis, and other chronic obstructive pulmonary disease
Diabetes	Diabetes mellitus
Gallbladder disorders	Cholethiasis and other disorders of gallbladder
Heart disease	Diseases of the heart
HIV disease	Human immunodeficiency virus (HIV) disease
Homicide	Assault (homicide)
Hypertension	Essential (primary) hypertension and hypertensive renal disease
Kidney disease	Nephritis, nephrotic syndrome, and nephrosis
Kidney infection	Infections of kidney

* World Health Organization. International Statistical Classification of Diseases and Related Health Problems, Tenth Revision (ICD-10). Geneva: World Health Organization, 1992. Available at http://www.who.int/classifications/icd/en/. Accessed April 15, 2014.

Legal intervention*	Physical or other force used by police or other law-enforcing agents, including military on duty, in the course of arresting or attempting to arrest lawbreakers, suppressing disturbances, maintaining order, and other legal action. Includes legal execution and excludes citizen arrest
Pelvic inflammatory diseases	Inflammatory diseases of female pelvic organs
Perinatal conditions	Certain conditions originating in the perinatal period
Pneumonitis	Pneumonitis due to solids and liquids
Pregnancy complications	Pregnancy, childbirth, and the puerperium
Stroke	Cerebrovascular diseases
Suicide	Intentional self-harm
Accidental injuries	Accidents (unintentional injuries)

Table 25. Women Top 10 Cancer Sites, 2010. United States*† Rates per 100,000‡

	Caucasian	African American	Asian/Pacific Islander §	American-Indian Alaska-Native §	Hispanic §‖
1	Female Breast 119.5	Female Breast 117.2	Female Breast 85.8	Female Breast 61.2	Female Breast 86.1
2	Lung and Bronchus 53.8	Lung and Bronchus 50.0	Colon and Rectum 28.5	Lung and Bronchus 36.2	Colon and Rectum 29.4
3	Colon and Rectum 34.4	Colon and Rectum 42.6	Lung and Bronchus 27.1	Colon and Rectum 27.0	Lung and Bronchus 25.0
4	Corpus and Uterus, NOS 25.2	Corpus and Uterus, NOS 23.4	Thyroid 20.1	Corpus and Uterus, NOS 15.6	Corpus and Uterus, NOS 20.0
5	Thyroid 20.9	Pancreas 13.6	Corpus and Uterus, NOS 17.7	Kidney and Renal Pelvis 11.8	Thyroid 19.0
6	Melanomas of the Skin 17.6	Thyroid 12.4	Non-Hodgkin Lymphoma 10.1	Non-Hodgkin Lymphoma 9.2	Non-Hodgkin Lymphoma 14.5
7	Non-Hodgkin Lymphoma 16.2	Kidney and Renal Pelvis 12.1	Pancreas 8.7	Thyroid 8.4	Kidney and Renal Pelvis 11.0
8	Ovary 11.8	Non-Hodgkin Lymphoma 11.7	Ovary 8.6	Ovary 7.8	Ovary 10.3
9	Kidney and Renal Pelvis 10.8	Myeloma 10.0	Stomach 8.3	Pancreas 7.5	Pancreas 10.0
10	Pancreas 10.3	Cervix 9.8	Liver & Intrahepatic Bile Duct 7.9	Leukemia 6.6	Cervix 9.6

US Cancer Statistics Working Group. United States Cancer Statistics: 1999–2010: US Department of Health and Human Services, CDC and National Cancer Institute; 2013.

Notes

* Data are from selected statewide and metropolitan area cancer registries that meet the data quality criteria for all invasive cancer sites combined. See registry-specific data quality information. Rates cover approximately 97 percent of the US population.

† Excludes basal and squamous cell carcinomas of the skin except when these occur on the skin of the genital organs, and in situ cancers except urinary bladder.

‡ Rates are age-adjusted to the 2000 US standard population (19 age groups—Census P25–1130).

§ Data for specified racial or ethnic populations other than white and black should be interpreted with caution.

|| Hispanic origin is not mutually exclusive from race categories (white, black, Asian/Pacific Islander, American Indian/Alaska Native).

~ Rates are suppressed and not ranked if case counts are fewer than 16 or if the population of the specific category (race, ethnicity) is less than 50,000.

Confidence interval (CI): Range of values for a rate that will include the true value of the rate a given percentage of the time. Example: 95 percent CI includes the true value of the rate 95 percent of the time.

Men Leading Causes of Death

The information contained in the following eight tables was obtained from HHS, CDC, and NCHS. The tables have been modified.

Table 26. Leading Causes of Death: Males in United States, 2010

Caucasian	%*	African American	%*
1) Heart disease	25.1	1) Heart disease	24.1
2) Cancer	24.6	2) Cancer	23.3
3) Unintentional injuries	6.2	3) Unintentional injuries	5.5
4) Chronic lower resp. diseases	5.7	4) Stroke	4.8
5) Stroke	4.1	5) Homicide	4.6
6) Diabetes	2.7	6) Diabetes	3.9
7) Suicide	2.6	7) Chronic lower resp. diseases	3.1
8) Alzheimer's disease	2.2	8) Kidney disease	2.8
9) Influenza / pneumonia	1.9	9) HIV disease	2.1
10) Kidney disease	1.9	10) Septicemia	1.8
Asian or Pacific Islander	%*	**Hispanic**	%*
1) Cancer	27.1	1) Cancer	20.7
2) Heart disease	23.5	2) Heart disease	20.6
3) Stroke	6.6	3) Unintentional injuries	9.5
4) Unintentional injuries	5	4) Stroke	4.2
5) Diabetes	3.5	5) Diabetes	4.2
6) Chronic lower resp. diseases	3.4	6) Chronic liver disease	3.9
7) Influenza and pneumonia	3.1	7) Homicide	3.1
8) Suicide	2.8	8) Chronic lower resp. diseases	2.7
9) Kidney disease	2	9) Suicide	2.7
10) Alzheimer's disease	1.3	10) Kidney	2.1

* Percent (%) represents total percentages of deaths.

Following Tables

Percentages represent total deaths in the age group due to the cause indicated. Numbers in parentheses indicate tied rankings. The white, black, American Indian/Alaska Native, and Asian/Pacific Islander race groups include persons of Hispanic and non-Hispanic origin who may be of any race. Some terms have been shortened from those used in the National Vital Statistics Report.

Refer to pages 146—147 for a listing of the shortened terms in the table and their full, unabridged equivalents used in the report.

Table 27. Men—Caucasian: Leading Cause of Death by Age Group—USA, 2010*

	Ages 15-19	20-24	25-34	35-44	45-54	55-64	65+
1	Accidental injuries 47.2%	Accidental injuries 49.5%	Accidental injuries 42.1%	Accidental injuries 26.1%	Cancer 22.7%	Cancer 32.4%	Heart disease 27.4%
2	Suicide 19.9%	Suicide 19.9%	Suicide 18.2%	Heart disease 16.1%	Heart disease 22.6%	Heart disease 24.9%	Cancer 25.0%
3	Homicide 9.9%	Homicide 8.4%	Heart disease 7.0%	Suicide 13.4%	Accidental injuries 12.6%	Accidental injuries 5.3%	Chronic lower resp. diseases 7.0%
4	Cancer 5.2%	Cancer 5.0%	Cancer 6.5%	Cancer 12.2%	Suicide 7.1%	Chronic lower resp. diseases 4.2%	Stroke 5.0%
5	Heart disease 2.9%	Heart disease 3.1%	Homicide 6.1%	Chronic liver disease 4.1%	Chronic liver disease 5.8%	Chronic liver disease 3.9%	Alzheimer's disease 3.2%
6	Birth defects 1.5%	Birth defects 1.0%	Chronic liver disease 1.2%	Homicide 2.7%	Diabetes 2.9%	Diabetes 3.6%	Diabetes 2.7%
7	Stroke 0.7%	Influenza and pneumonia 0.5%	Diabetes 1.0%	Diabetes 2.1%	Stroke 2.5%	Suicide 3.0%	Accidental injuries 2.6%

Table 28. Men—African American: Leading Cause of Death by Age Group—USA, 2010*

	Ages 15-19	20-24	25-34	35-44	45-54	55-64	65+
1	Homicide 50.4%	Homicide 49.2%	Homicide 35.1%	Heart disease 20.6%	Heart disease 26.6%	Cancer 29.9%	Cancer 27.4%
2	Accidental injuries 22.3%	Accidental injuries 20.0%	Accidental injuries 19.5%	Accidental injuries 13.7%	Cancer 21.1%	Heart disease 26.3%	Heart disease 27.1%
3	Suicide 6.7%	Suicide 8.4%	Heart disease 9.5%	Homicide 11.2%	Accidental injuries 8.1%	Stroke 5.0%	Stroke 5.7%
4	Heart disease 3.6%	Heart disease 4.5%	Suicide 7.1%	Cancer 9.8%	HIV disease 5.6%	Diabetes 4.4%	Chronic lower resp. diseases 4.5%
5	Cancer 2.9%	HIV disease 4.5%	HIV disease 8.1%	Stroke 4.7%	Accidental injuries 4.1%	Diabetes 4.3%	Chronic lower resp. diseases 4.3%
6	Birth defects 1.8%	HIV disease 1.9%	Cancer 4.2%	Suicide 4.4%	Diabetes 4.1%	Kidney disease 2.8%	Kidney disease 3.6%
7	Anemia 1.1%	Anemia 1.1%	Diabetes 1.9%	Homicide 2.8%	Chronic lower resp. diseases 2.6%	Influenza and pneumonia 2.2%	Accidental injuries 2.1%

Table 29. Men—Asian or Pacific Islander: Leading Cause of Death by Age Group—USA, 2010*

	Ages 15-19	20-24	25-34	35-44	45-54	55-64	65+
1	Accidental injuries 38.1%	Accidental injuries 35.1%	Accidental injuries 28.5%	Cancer 21.8%	Cancer 31.5%	Cancer 37.6%	Heart disease 26.4%
2	Suicide 21.6%	Suicide 27.2%	Suicide 21.6%	Heart disease 19.0%	Heart disease 23.0%	Heart disease 23.0%	Cancer 26.0%
3	Homicide 10.8%	Cancer 9.8%	Cancer 12.3%	Accidental injuries 13.0%	Stroke 6.9%	Stroke 6.1%	Stroke 7.3%
4	Cancer 9.1%	Homicide 8.7%	Heart disease 10.1%	Suicide 11.7%	Accidental injuries 6.8%	Diabetes 4.9%	Chronic lower resp. diseases 4.7%
5	Heart disease 4.0%	Heart disease 5.2%	Homicide 6.7%	Stroke 6.2%	Suicide 5.6%	Accidental injuries 3.7%	Influenza and pneumonia 4.1%
6	Birth defects 3.4%	Stroke 0.8% *** Birth defects 0.8%	Stroke 1.7%	Homicide 3.7%	Diabetes 3.5%	Suicide 2.7%	Diabetes 3.7%
7	Influenza and pneumonia 2.3%	***	Birth defects 1.5%	Chronic liver disease 3.0%	Chronic liver disease 3.1%	Chronic liver disease 2.3%	Accidental injuries 2.5%

Table 30. Men—Hispanic: Leading Cause of Death by Age Group—USA, 2010*

	Ages 15-19	20-24	25-34	35-44	45-54	55-64	65+
1	Accidental injuries 35.4%	Accidental injuries 43.1%	Accidental injuries 35.6%	Accidental injuries 24.7%	Cancer 19.8%	Cancer 27.7%	Heart disease 26.6%
2	Homicide 29.2%	Homicide 21.9%	Homicide 16.6%	Heart disease 12.7%	Heart disease 18.8%	Heart disease 22.8%	Cancer 24.4%
3	Suicide 13.6%	Suicide 11.3%	Cancer 11.3%	Accidental injuries 11.7%	Chronic liver disease 7.3%	Stroke 5.5%	Diabetes 6.3%
4	Cancer 5.9%	Cancer 7.1%	Suicide 7.5%	Chronic liver disease 9.8%	Diabetes 6.1%	Diabetes 5.1%	Stroke 4.8%
5	Heart disease 2.6%	Heart disease 2.5%	Heart disease 6.6%	Chronic liver disease 6.7%	Stoke 4.1%	Accidental injuries 5.4%	Chronic lower resp. diseases 4.4%
6	Birth defects 0.9%	HIV disease 2.4%	Homicide 6.1%	Diabetes 3.9%	Stroke 3.9%	Kidney disease 2.9%	Chronic lower resp. diseases 3.3%
7	HIV disease 0.8%	Chronic liver disease 2.1%	HIV disease 4.2%	Suicide 3.6%	Viral hepatitis 2.3%	Influenza and pneumonia 2.9%	Kidney disease 2.7%

Short and Full Terms for Leading Causes of Death (Males)

Some terms in the leading causes of death tables have been shortened from those used in the National Vital Statistics Report. Below is a listing of the shortened terms used in the table and their full, unabridged equivalents used in the report.

Short Terms	Full Terms
Aortic aneurism	Aortic aneurism and dissection
Benign neoplasms	In situ neoplasms and neoplasms of uncertain or unknown behavior
Birth defects	Congenital malformations, deformations and chromosomal abnormalities
Bronchitis	Acute bronchitis and bronchiolitis
Cancer	Malignant neoplasms
C. difficile infection	Enter colitis due to clostridium
Chronic liver disease	Chronic liver disease and cirrhosis
Chronic lower– respiratory diseases	Includes bronchitis, emphysema, asthma, bronchiectasis, and other chronic obstructive pulmonary disease
Diabetes	Diabetes mellitus
Gallbladder disorders	Cholethiasis and other disorders of gallbladder
Heart disease	Diseases of the heart
HIV disease	Human immunodeficiency virus (HIV) disease
Homicide	Assault (homicide)
Hypertension	Essential (primary) hypertension and hypertensive renal disease
Kidney disease	Nephritis, nephrotic syndrome, and nephrosis
Kidney infection	Infections of kidney

* World Health Organization. International statistical Classification of Diseases and Related Health Problems, Tenth Revision (ICD-10). Geneva: World Health Organization, 1992. Available at http://www.who.int/ classifications/icd/en/. Accessed April 15, 2010.

Legal Intervention* — Physical or other force used by police or other law-enforcing agents, including military on duty, in the course of arresting or attempting to arrest lawbreakers, suppressing disturbances, maintaining order, and other legal action. Includes legal execution and excludes citizen arrest.

Medical and surgical– care complications — Complications of medical and surgical care

Operations of war — Operations of War and their Sequelae

Perinatal conditions — Certain conditions originating in the perinatal period

Pneumonitis — Pneumonitis due to solids and liquids

Stroke — Cerebrovascular diseases

Suicide — Intentional self-harm

Accidental injuries — Accidents (unintentional injuries)

Table 31. Men Top 10 Cancer Sites: 2010, United States *† Rates per 100,000 ‡

	Caucasian	African American	Asian/Pacific Islander §	American Indian Alaska Native §	Hispanic §||
1	Prostate 115.6	Prostate 192.9	Prostate 63.7	Prostate 66.8	Prostate 104.8
2	Lung and Bronchus 73.7	Lung and Bronchus 86.8	Lung and Bronchus 46.1	Lung and Bronchus 49.7	Lung and Bronchus 42.1
3	Colon and Rectum 45.2	Colon and Rectum 56.9	Colon and Rectum 38.5	Colon and Rectum 32.1	Colon and Rectum 41.7
4	Urinary Bladder 37.2	Kidney and Renal Pelvis 22.2	Liver & Intrahep. Bile Duct 19.7	Kidney and Renal Pelvis 19.1	Non-Hodgkin Lymphoma 19.8
5	Melanomas of the Skin 26.8	Urinary Bladder 18.4	Urinary Bladder 15.2	Urinary Bladder 13.4	Kidney and Renal Pelvis 19.7
6	Non-Hodgkin Lymphoma 23.0	Non-Hodgkin Lymphoma 16.9	Non-Hodgkin Lymphoma 15.1	Non-Hodgkin Lymphoma 12.6	Liver & Intrahep. Bile Duct 19.4
7	Kidney and Renal Pelvis 20.6	Pancreas 16.5	Stomach 14.5	Liver & Intrahep. Bile Duct 11.8	Urinary Bladder 19.0
8	Oral Cavity and Pharynx 16.5	Liver & Intrahep. Bile Duct 15.0	Oral Cavity and Pharynx 10.8	Oral Cavity and Pharynx 10.2	Stomach 13.4
9	Leukemia 16.4	Oral Cavity and Pharynx 14.2	Kidney and Renal Pelvis 10.7	Pancreas 7.8	Leukemia 12.2
10	Pancreas 13.3	Stomach 14.0	Pancreas 9.3	Stomach 7.7	Pancreas 11.6

US Cancer Statistics Working Group. United States Cancer Statistics: 1999–2010 Incidence and Mortality Web-Based Report. Atlanta: US Department of Health and Human Services, Centers for Disease Control and Prevention and National Cancer Institute, 2013.

Notes

* Data are from selected statewide and metropolitan area cancer registries that meet the data quality criteria for all invasive cancer sites combined. See registry-specific data quality information. Rates cover approximately 97 percent of the US population.

† Excludes basal and squamous cell carcinomas of the skin except when these occur on the skin of the genital organs, and in situ cancers except urinary bladder.

‡ Rates are age-adjusted to the 2000 US standard population (19 age groups—Census P25-1130).

§ Data for specified racial or ethnic populations other than white and black should be interpreted with caution. See Technical Notes.

‖ Hispanic origin is not mutually exclusive from race categories (white, black, Asian/Pacific Islander, American Indian/Alaska Native).

~ Rates are suppressed and not ranked if case counts are fewer than 16 or if the population of the specific category (race, ethnicity) is less than 50,000.

Confidence interval (CI): Range of values for a rate that will include the true value of the rate a given percentage of the time. Example: 95 percent CI includes the true value of the rate 95 percent of the time.

Conclusion

Nutrients affect every aspect of your health. Your health affects every aspect of your life. Every few years a new wonder-diet goes viral and multitudes of "experts" flood the internet with blogs and forums telling the world that this is the diet we have all been searching for (until the next one comes along). They blame entire food groups for all that ills mankind in order to push their agenda. There are risks and benefits associated with virtually everything that you eat. Faux diets mislead others by focusing only on the risks associated with one food group, and the benefits associated with another. Their extreme measures and misleading information may cause more long-term harm than short-term good.

There are no miracle pills or miracle foods for long-term health. In addition, there is no such thing as the perfect diet. With that said, regardless of the dietary path that you choose, optimum health and performance begins at the cellular level. Give your cells the proper balance of nutrients they need to flourish. In turn, they will optimize your strength, energy, and focus throughout your life. Your body is a complex and unique structure. As the builders, your cells need the right combination of tools and raw materials to construct and maintain that complex and unique structure called *you*. Having too many or too few tools or materials than your cells require will impede their ability to perform at their peak.

Health and nutrition are extremely comprehensive, yet they are also fairly simple once you have objective facts versus subjective assertions. The information you have just read is based on peer-reviewed, scientifically tested data from a multitude of nations. This mitigates the potential for group-think. In other words, groups of like-minded individuals have not conspired to sell you a product or lifestyle. Numerous, credible, independent studies around the world have simply drawn similar conclusions that do not come and go with the prevailing winds. These are basic, often overlooked, facts that can be used to forge a long-term foundation of cellular health. It is doable, and more importantly, it is sustainable.

The focus is not on what to avoid at all cost, or to fear. The focus is not on extreme measures or dramatic lifestyle changes. The focus is on basic, key nutrient balance—and how anyone, at any level of fitness, can achieve it. Runners, weightlifters, cyclists, and couch potatoes alike can improve their health, focus, immunity, healing, and energy by reversing nutrient deficiencies and removing nutrient excess.

Improving cellular health through nutrient balance can also reduce dependency on costly prescription drugs and healthcare procedures. As with many people who suffer from asthma, I often kept three rescue inhalers strategically placed in my home, vehicle, and workplace. Now, I only have one—and I barely use it. If I forget to bring it home from work, I no longer suffer from the anxiety of not having it with me. Moreover, I no longer require preventive inhalers which were quite expensive for me and my insurance carrier. It is possible for individuals to reduce or even stop periodic medical treatments by attaining their proper nutrient balance. Nevertheless, do not attempt to do so without medical supervision.

There is far more nutrient-based information available than contained within these pages. With that said, the information you have just read addresses several of the most commonly overlooked or misdiagnosed nutrient deficiencies in industrialized nations. Resolving them affords you the biggest health gains for the smallest investments.

Consistency and balance are essential. Do not megadose on any vitamin or mineral, especially over an extended period. It takes years to develop nutrient deficiencies. Taking moderate doses over time can reverse nutrient deficiencies without injuring your organs, brain, and nervous system. Always think of your health in terms of years and decades instead of days or weeks. If you have been megadosing on supplements, gradually reduce the dosages and frequency (if needed) over a two to four week period. Be patient and determined.

I encourage you to consider testing the information contained here for at least thirty days. If you need supplementation to meet your nutrient requirements, purchase three 7-day pill containers. Buy different colors for the morning, noon, and evening. Prefill all three with supplements each week. Be creative. Stagger your supplements in a manner that fits your schedule. Remember, skipping a day or two with most supplements can actually be beneficial.

As a reminder, many people are moderately deficient in zinc, magnesium, potassium, and vitamin D. Regaining recommended levels of these nutrients alone—coupled with a high-quality multivitamin—can yield very quick and noticeable results. Always choose quality supplements over quantity.

This is your opportunity to improve your health and vitality at the cellular level. This is your opportunity to offer your cells the environment they need to build and maintain an even stronger and healthier you. Give yourself the gift of optimum cellular performance. Be patient. Be consistent. Most importantly, be well.

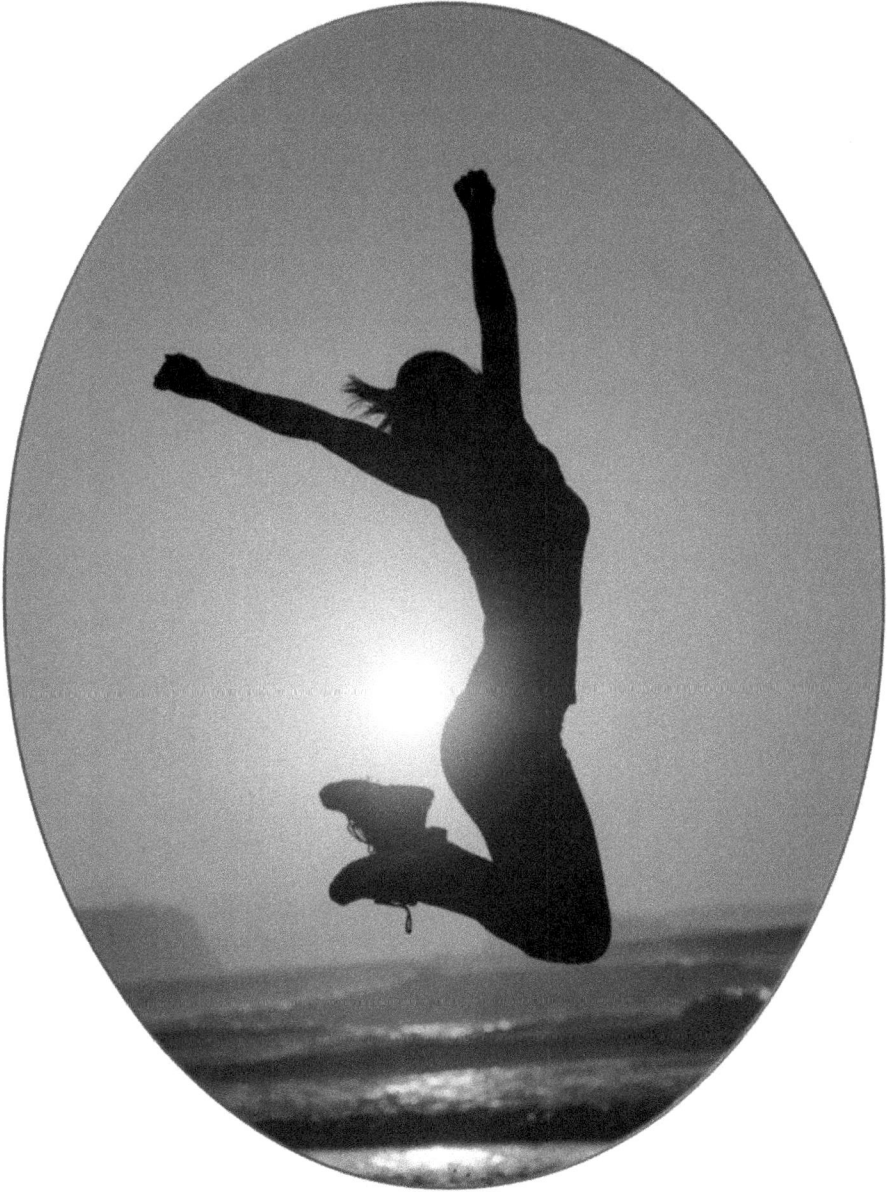

What's next???

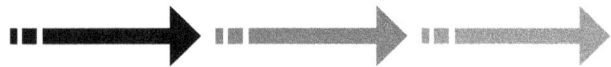

It's Not the Cans—For
Healthier Kids and Teens

Children's health greatly influences how they will function for their entire lives. Each phase of their life requires a stage-specific nutritional balance to reach his or her fullest potential.

According to the CDC, in the past, type 2 diabetes was most common in people over age forty-five. But now more young people, even children, have the disease because many are overweight or obese.

It's Not the Cans—For Healthier Kids and Teens (coming soon) will address the nutritional needs for leaner, healthier children and teens. In it, we will discuss nutrition for a healthier brain (improved learning), body (improved energy and weight management), and immune system (improved defense against illness and injury). We will also discuss preventive measures to reduce the risk of developing life-threatening illnesses such as diabetes and heart disease when they become adults.

It's Not the Cans (online)

Visit www.notthecans.com for additional nutrient information and preferred products. You will also find links to external websites that focus on nutrition and health. Preferred product recommendations are based on products that yield a high level of nutritional quality for the price. Although you will be able to make purchases on our website, you are encouraged to support your local vitamin store.

Glossary

Adequate Intake (AI) levels are established when there is not enough documented evidence to develop an RDA. AI is set at a level assumed to ensure nutritional adequacy. AI is based on observed intakes of the nutrient by a group of healthy persons.

Bioavailability is a term used to identify the ease or difficulty of a nutrient to absorb into your system. A high bioavailability means you will absorb more of the nutrient.

Buffering a substance reduces its potential to irritate your digestive system with symptoms such as nausea or diarrhea. Buffering will make a substance either less alkaline or less acidic (see pH Balance).

Chelation is a method of binding a substance to a protein to increase its bioavailability. Binding a substance to a protein greatly increases its absorption rate.

Dietary reference intakes (DRIs) are based on multiple reference values; Adequate Intake (AI), Recommended Dietary Allowance (RDA), Tolerable Upper Intake Level (UL).

Estimated Average Requirement (EAR) is the amount of a nutrient that is estimated to meet the requirement of half of all healthy individuals in the population

Gastrointestinal (GI) Transit Time is the amount of time required for food to pass through to your stool, which is 1.5–3 days on average. High-protein meals travel at a slower pace allowing the protein to be absorbed more fully. Foods you eat are not expelled in the same order that you eat them. Some food elements are pushed past others.

Megadose far exceeds required amounts of vitamins, minerals, or other supplements. Megadosing on supplements can result in irreversible internal damage and premature death.

Minerals are primarily used to build strong bones and teeth, regulate fluid inside and outside cells, create energy, and transfer electrical signals though your nervous system.

Nutrient balance, for the purposes of this discussion, is the proper level, ratio, and range of synergetic nutrients needed to produce optimum cellular performance.

pH Balance occurs when the pH level of a substance equals 7, making it neither acidic nor alkaline. A pH number from 0 to14 indicates how acidic or alkaline a substance is. Anything above 7 is alkaline, and anything below 7 is acid. Water has a pH level of 7, which is neutral. It has the same amount of acids and alkalis, which balance each other out. When you're thinking about liquids in terms of their pH levels, going up or down one number on the scale represents a tenfold change in the acidity or alkaline nature of a liquid. For example, the pH level of milk is around 6. Because the pH level of water is 7, milk is 10 times more acidic than water.

Recommended Dietary Allowance (RDA) is the average daily level of intake sufficient to meet the nutrient requirements of nearly all (97–98 percent) healthy individuals.

Tolerable Upper Intake Level (UL) is the maximum daily intake unlikely to cause harm.

Vitamins (Fat-Soluble) are ingested from animal fats, butter, vegetable oils, dairy, fish, and liver. Your body is very effective at storing these vitamins in your liver and fatty tissues for future use. If you regularly consume more than you need (megadose), some fat-soluble vitamins can damage your organs, nervous system, and brain. Fat-soluble vitamins remain available even after foods containing them are cooked (see *Nutrient Retention*). They absorb best with meals containing healthy fats (e.g., flaxseed, olive oil, eggs, avocados, lake herring, lake trout, mackerel, wild salmon, sardines, and tuna).
Fat-soluble vitamins are vitamins A, D, E, and K.

Vitamins (Water-Soluble) are mainly sourced from fruits, vegetables, and grains and are not as resilient to heat as fat-soluble vitamins. Water-soluble vitamins are not stored very long and need to be replenished more frequently. Excess is primarily excreted via your urine.

About the Author

Born and raised on the south side of Chicago, Bryant Lusk displayed a natural affinity for science and technology. As a young man, he served four years of active military duty in the US Air Force within the field of Avionics. Despite his humble beginnings, Bryant excelled at resolving extremely technical issues while working at Motorola Inc., and Raytheon TSC. Bryant's passion to serve a greater purpose led him to the Federal Aviation Administration (FAA).

Nearly thirty years of experience in science and technology, coupled with a strong desire to protect others motivated Bryant to write this book. He currently resides in Bellevue Washington.

"I measure success by the number of people that I affect in a positive and meaningful way."

— Bryant Lusk

www.ingramcontent.com/pod-product-compliance
Lightning Source LLC
Chambersburg PA
CBHW081415270326
41931CB00015B/3286